OWN YOUR CALM

Conceived, designed, and produced by
The Bright Press,
an imprint of the Quarto Group,
1 Triptych Place, London SE1 9SH,
United Kingdom
T (0)20 7700 6700
www.Quarto.com

ISBN: 978-1-4197-8632-7

Author: Jo Usmar

For The Bright Press
Publisher: James Evans
Editorial Director: Isheeta Mustafi
Art Director: Emily Nazer
Managing Editor: Lucy Tipton
Editor: Ellie Stores
Design: Marcia Pedraza Sierra

Published in 2026 by Abrams, an imprint of ABRAMS.

For Abrams
Editor: Juliet Dore
Design Manager: Danielle Youngsmith
Managing Editor: Grace Ball
Production Manager: Larry Pakarek

Printed and bound in Pontian, Johor, Malaysia
PC/11/2025

ABRAMS is represented in the UK and Europe by Abrams & Chronicle Books, 22-24 Ely Place, London EC1N 6TE and Média-Participations, 57 rue Gaston Tessier, 75166 Paris, France.
www.abramsandchronicle.co.uk and www.mediaparticipations.com
info@abramsandchronicle.co.uk

10 9 8 7 6 5 4 3 2 1

Abrams products are available at special discounts when purchased in quantity for premiums and promotions as well as fundraising or educational use. Special editions can also be created to specification. For details, contact specialsales@abramsbooks.com or the address below.

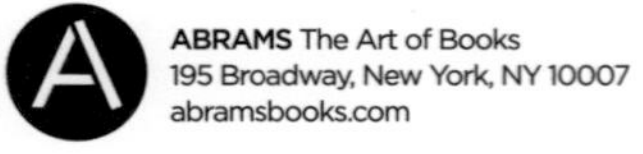

ABRAMS The Art of Books
195 Broadway, New York, NY 10007
abramsbooks.com

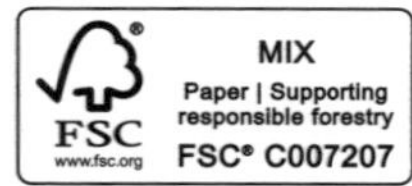

OWN YOUR CALM

A Guided Journal for
Overcoming Anxiety

JO USMAR

Abrams, New York

Contents

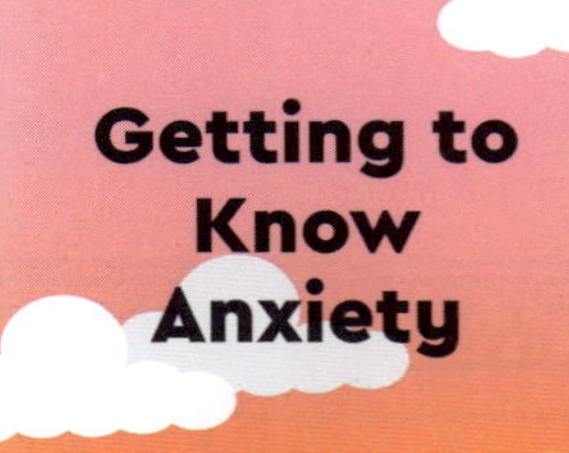

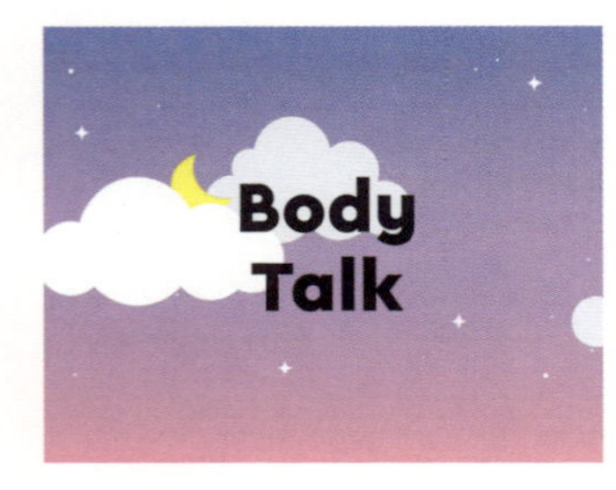

Introduction

Thank you so much for picking up this book. I'm glad it caught your eye—the thought of owning your calm speaks to me too. It has never felt more necessary to make time to take a breath, a beat, a moment. To tune out the noise of the world and tune back into ourselves.

What does it mean to be calm? It is when we feel peaceful and clearheaded. It's a steady self-belief that says: "I can do this" or "I can cope." When we feel this way, even a crisis won't shake us. We'll manage it with coolness and composure. Yet, that's not always how life works. As humans, we're wired to experience the full spectrum of emotions. Like it or not, we don't get to cherry-pick the good stuff. Anxiety, fear, stress—they're part of the package and are totally normal. However, when pressure builds, those feelings can take over, causing our rational, decision-making, and problem-solving brain to retreat—affecting how we feel physically and mentally, and how we respond. This can create negative cycles that are hard to break.

Here's the good news: calm *is* within reach. And you're much more capable than you think you are. This journal is your toolkit for changing how you respond to stress by learning to meet it differently. Owning your calm means recognizing that anxiety isn't permanent. It does pass—and you *can* stop things from spiraling. It's about spotting unhelpful patterns, trusting in your resilience, being self-compassionate, and finding optimism in the everyday.

You've got this.

Jo Usmar

(P.S. If you think you may have an anxiety disorder, please do speak to your doctor—specialist support can make a huge difference.)

How to Get the Most from This Journal

Inside, you'll find simple journal prompts to help you reflect on how anxiety impacts your mood, thoughts, body, and behavior—and begin to see how they're all connected.

Drawing on CBT techniques and mindfulness, the questions are designed to help you untangle worries, soften the sharp edge of self-doubt, and recognize self-defeating behavior. In doing so, you'll build a more compassionate, grounded perspective on whatever it is you're facing.

There are tracking pages to work through specific issues as well as to record your progress. Tracking is an incredibly effective way to recognize your triggers and recurring responses. It helps you to step back from anxious thoughts by giving time and space for processing, organizing, and regrouping. You'll also find practical advice, helpful facts, and anti-anxiety reminders throughout, guiding you through stressful moments.

This journal is divided into six parts, designed to be flexible. You can work through them in order, or simply dip in and out. Wherever you land, you'll find something to reflect on and take with you.

The first four parts explore how anxiety can show up in your mood, body, thoughts, and behavior, and offer practical tools to help interrupt the classic stress domino effect. Part Five focuses on the future, sharing timeless strategies for owning your calm in everyday life. In Part Six, you'll find a full year's worth of monthly trackers with space to set gentle intentions, notice how things unfold, and reflect on how things went.

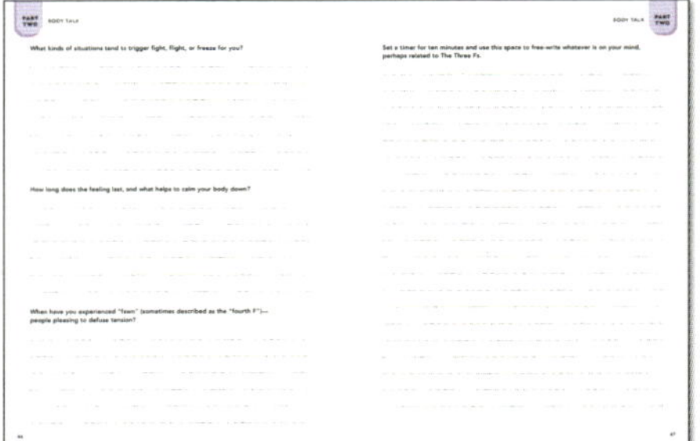

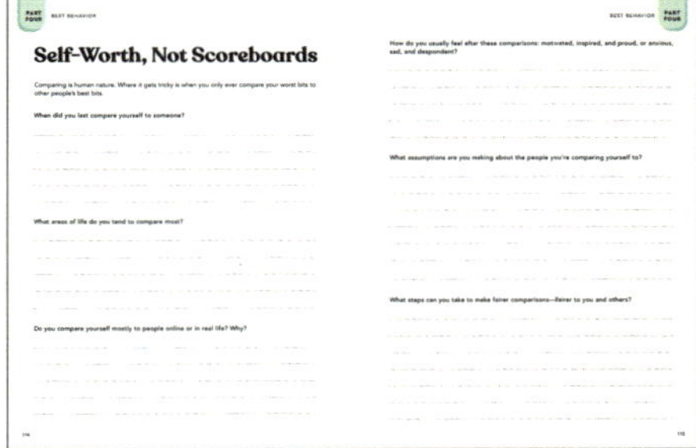

Journal prompts that you can find throughout the book

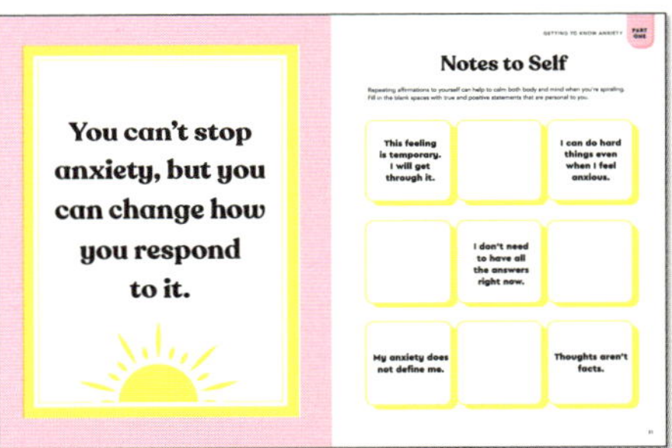

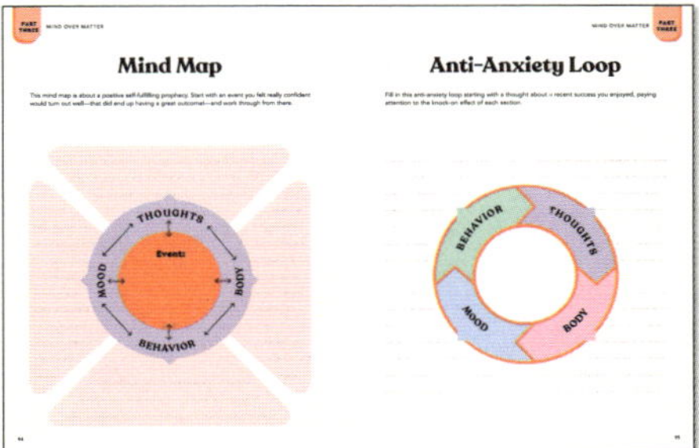

Practical exercises to help you work through your anxieties

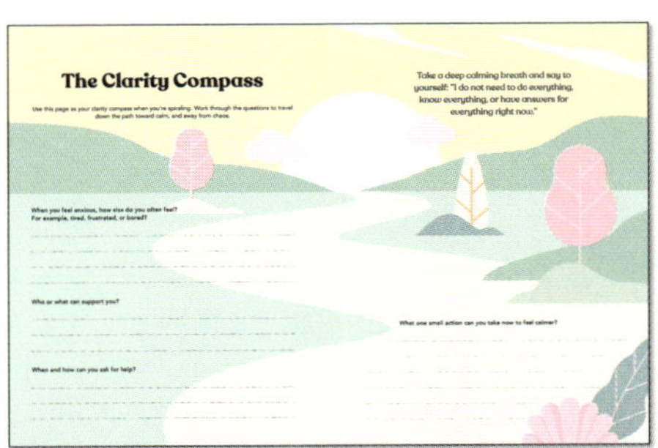

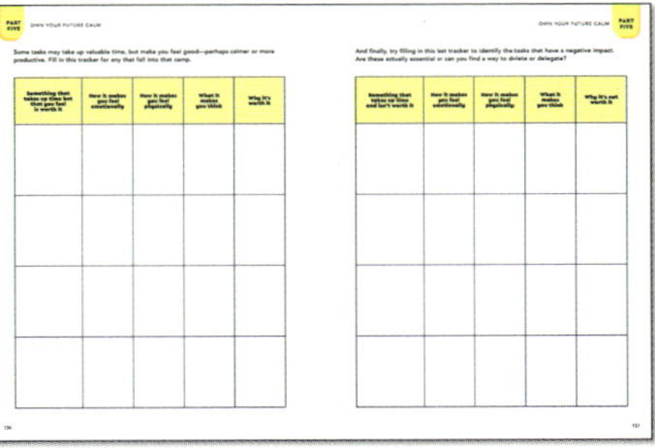

Part Five contains techniques and strategies for the future

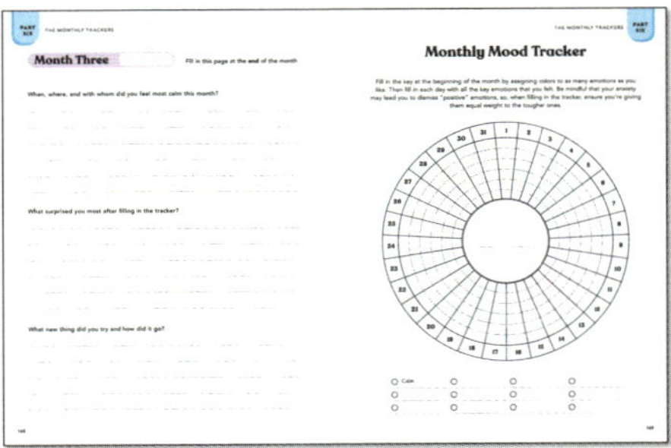

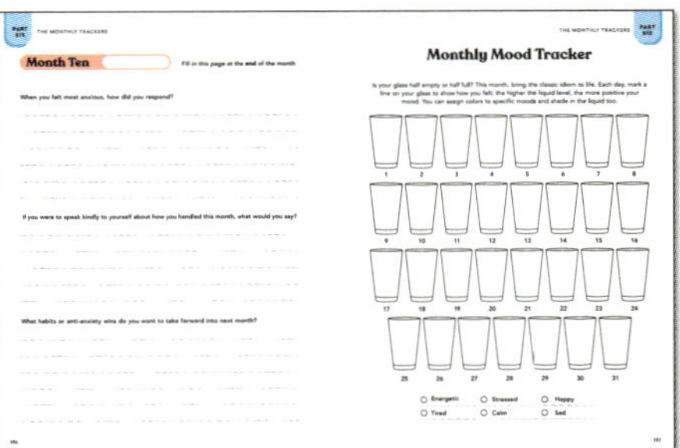

In Part Six, you'll find monthly trackers for a whole year

Name the Noise

Here, you'll find definitions of anxiety, stress, fear, panic, and worry. While these terms are often used interchangeably, for a deeper understanding of your personal response to events, it's essential to understand the subtle differences so you can learn how to limit their impact.

Anxiety

An anticipatory emotion triggered by persistent unease or the possibility of something going wrong. For instance, "I'm anxious about how X or Y might turn out."

Stress

Stress isn't an emotion, but a physical or mental response to pressure, so, "I'm stressed about work" rather than, "I'm anxious about the possible repercussions if work goes wrong."

Fear

An emotion, fear is our built-in threat-detector. It warns us about known threats or dangers. For example, "I fear X or Y happening."

Panic

The most severe form of anxiety or fear, panic is a response to threats in the immediate moment, like, "I feel I am in danger right now."

Worry

The repetitive, often snowballing thought processes that can fuel anxiety, stress, and fear, as well as be fueled by them, such as, "What if…?"

Note down some recent challenging situations and check which boxes ring true for your experience at the time. Name that noise!

Situation	Anxiety	Stress	Fear	Panic	Worry

PART ONE

Getting to Know Anxiety

Everyone experiences anxiety differently. Understanding how it affects you personally will open up new ways to manage symptoms, make meaningful changes, and feel calmer.

How Anxiety Affects You

Why do you feel you need to better own your calm?

How much of an impact does anxiety have on your life?

What do you wish people knew about you that anxiety stops you from showing?

How does your anxiety show you what you care deeply about?

What anxiety-led stories about yourself have you started to believe?

Choose a color that you think fits each sentence best and then describe why you chose them.

- ◯ What anxiety feels like
- ◯ What calm feels like
- ◯ What an average day feels like
- ◯ What I want an average day to feel like

The House of Anxiety

Have you felt worried recently? Start at the top floor, then follow the instructions and walk these worries "downstairs," to discover the foundational fears that they're based on.

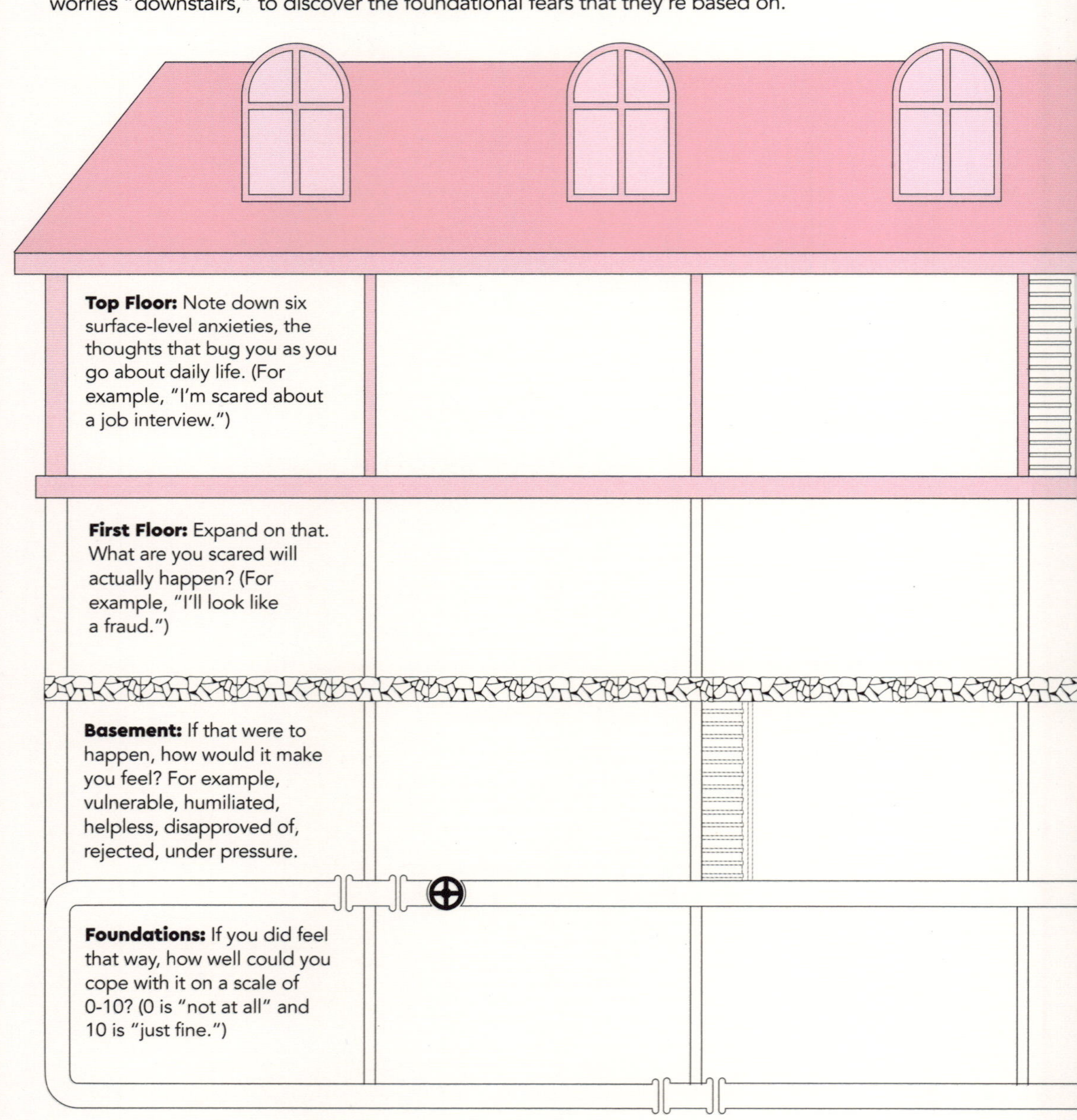

Top Floor: Note down six surface-level anxieties, the thoughts that bug you as you go about daily life. (For example, "I'm scared about a job interview.")

First Floor: Expand on that. What are you scared will actually happen? (For example, "I'll look like a fraud.")

Basement: If that were to happen, how would it make you feel? For example, vulnerable, humiliated, helpless, disapproved of, rejected, under pressure.

Foundations: If you did feel that way, how well could you cope with it on a scale of 0-10? (0 is "not at all" and 10 is "just fine.")

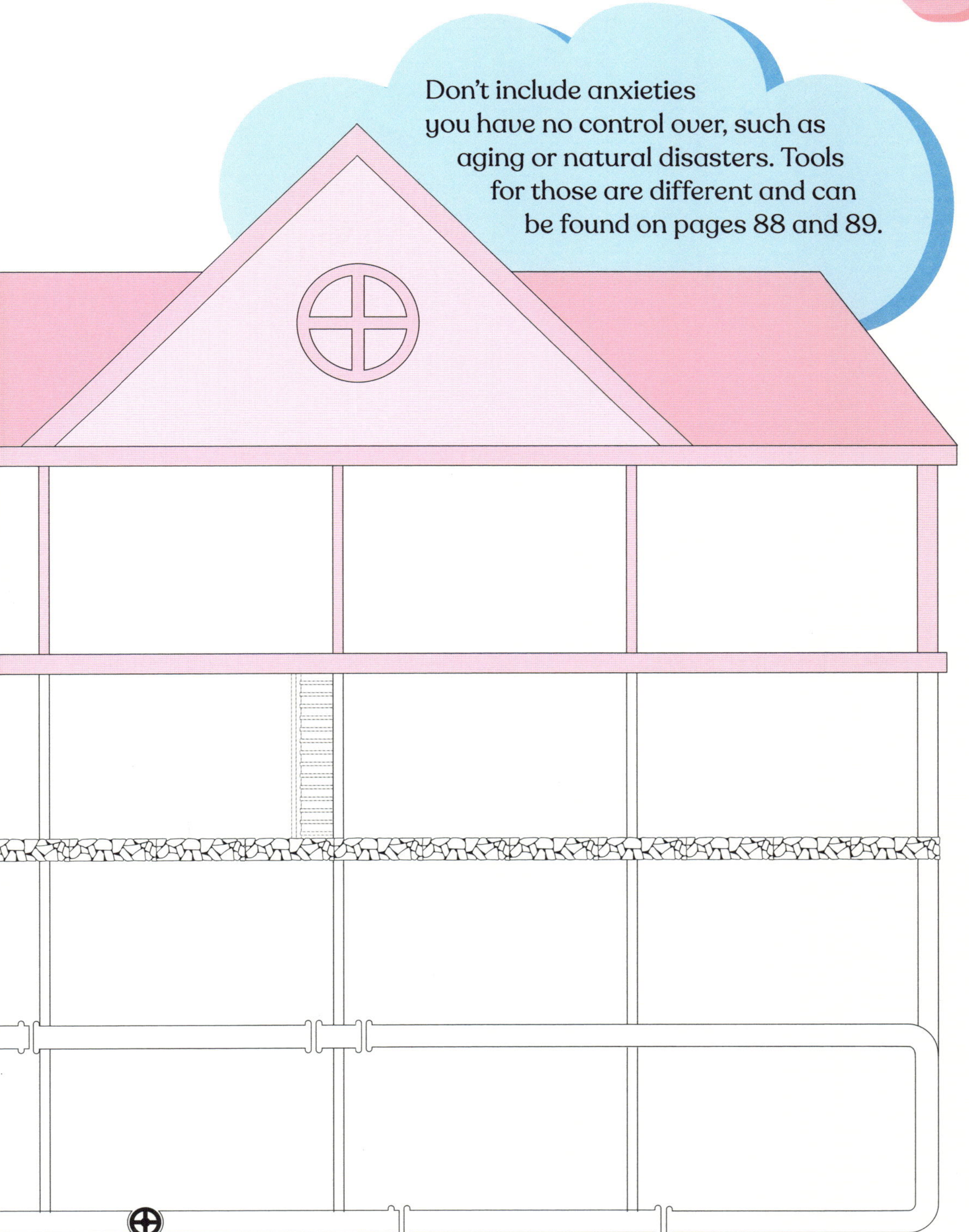
Don't include anxieties
you have no control over, such as
aging or natural disasters. Tools
for those are different and can
be found on pages 88 and 89.

After completing The House of Anxiety tracker, how do you feel about how you rated your ability to cope?

How would someone who loves you rate your ability to cope, and why? (Consider what skills or qualities they see in you.)

Set a 10 minute timer and free-write whatever you're feeling about getting to know your anxiety.

Mind Maps

Mind maps help show how your mood, thoughts, body, and behavior respond to an event, and how they affect one another. They break experiences into manageable parts, highlighting potential "interruption points" for change. In this first mind map, start with a recent event that triggered anxiety, then fill in the response boxes in any order.

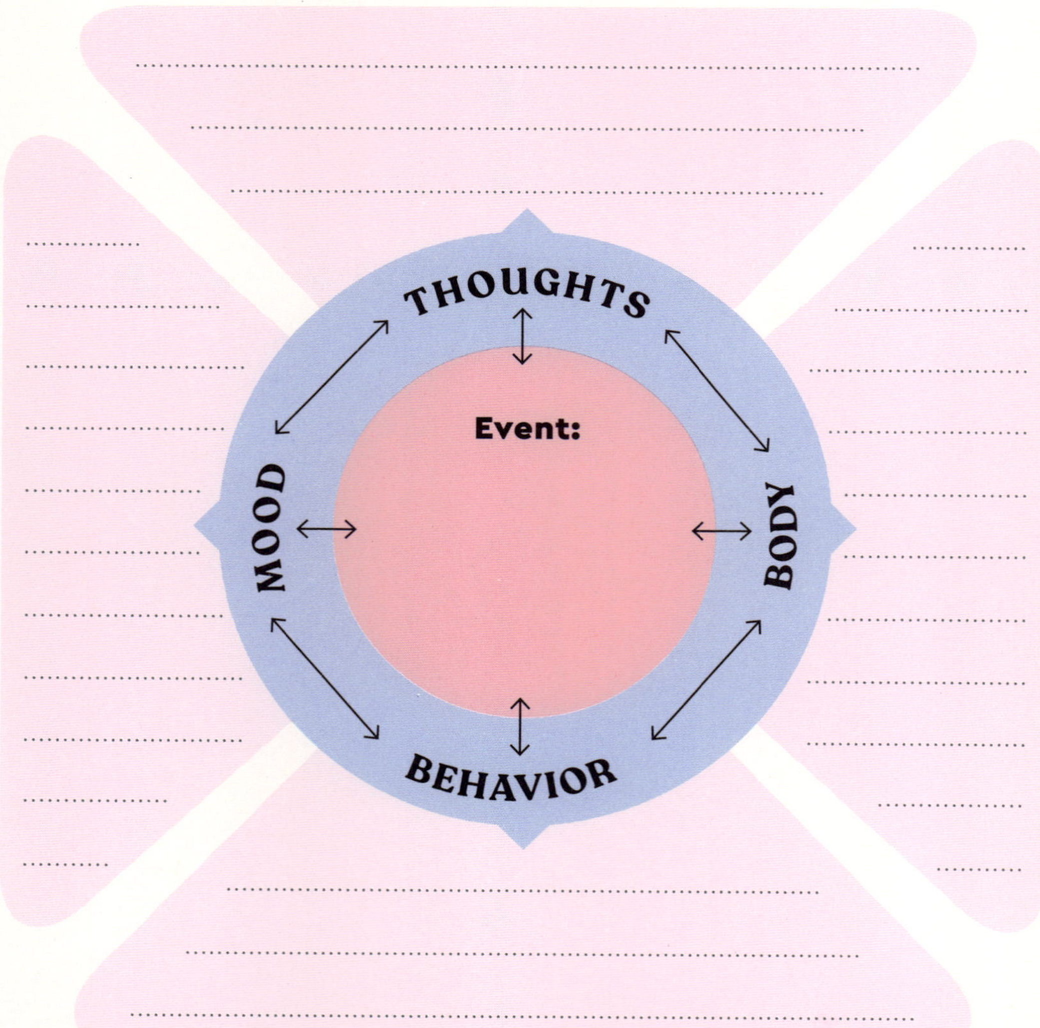

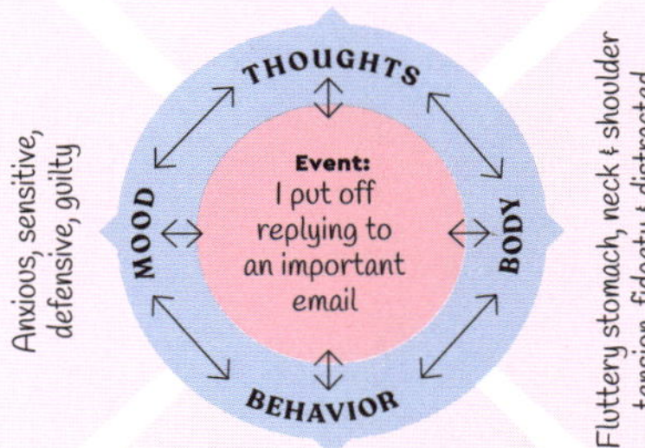

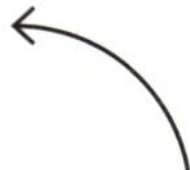

Use this as an example.

Do the same with the second mind map, using a more positive event as the jumping off point.

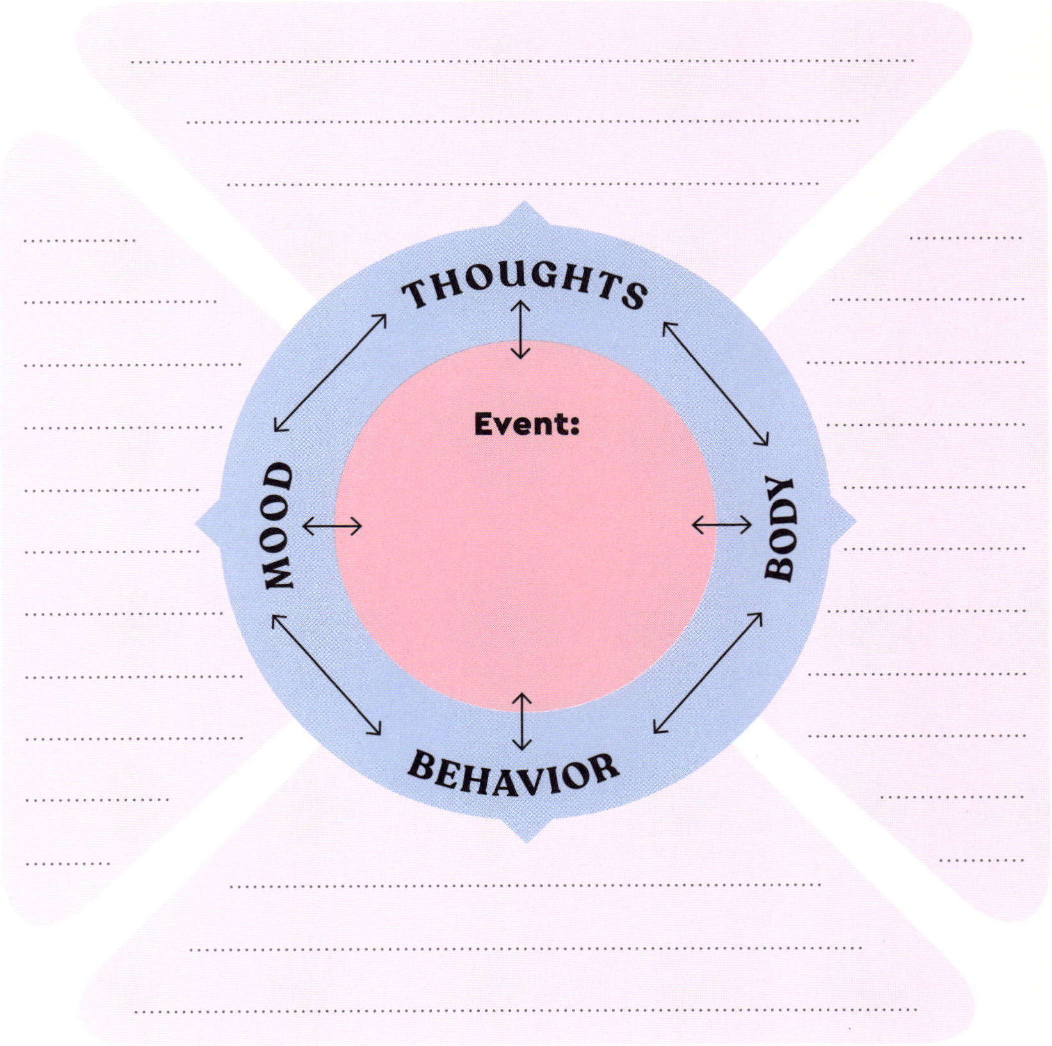

THOUGHTS

MOOD

Event:

BODY

BEHAVIOR

Anti-Anxiety Loops

When we feel low, it can lead to a chain reaction—an anxiety loop—where you end up worrying about your worry, and the negative domino effect escalates. The good news? It works just the same when we feel calm, leading to more grounded cycles of thoughts, behaviors, and physical responses.

BEHAVIOR

THOUGHTS

BODY

MOOD

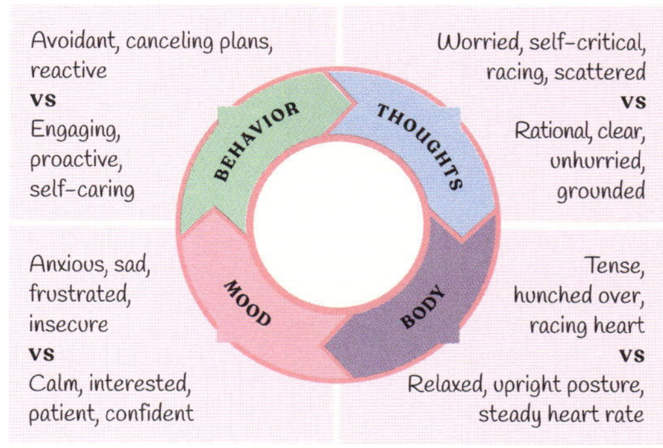

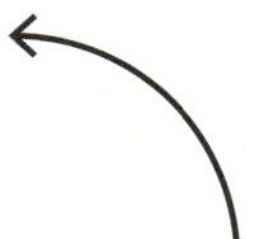

Fill in your own loops using examples of when you felt anxious and when you felt calm.

You can start at any point around the circle.

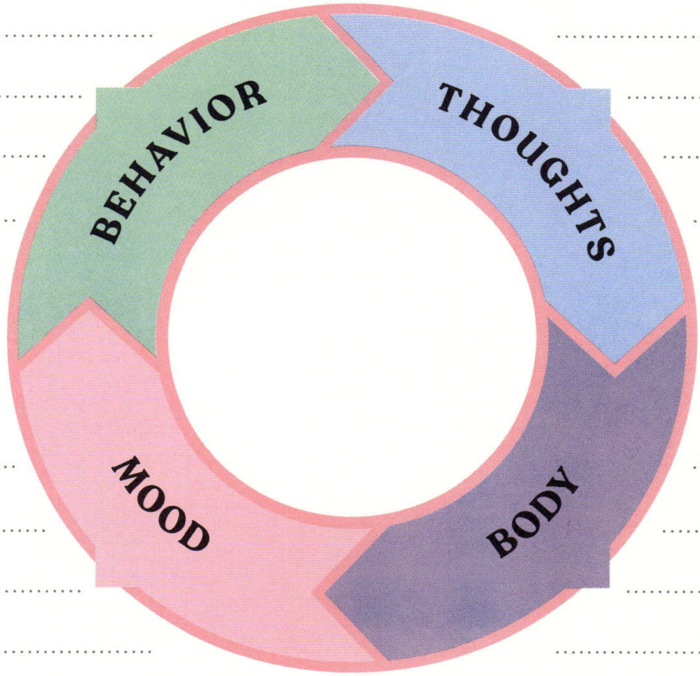

BEHAVIOR

THOUGHTS

MOOD

BODY

When anxiety hits, what do you notice first—your thoughts, body, behavior, or mood? Does one element feel "bigger" than the others?

Which element affects your daily life the most and why?

What do you think your anxiety might be trying to protect you from and why?

Do you get more stressed over internal pressure (what you're asking of yourself) or external pressure (what's being asked of you)?

Where might this anxiety have come from—perhaps family, friends, popular culture, social media, or a specific event?

Do you remember when it started?

Start tuning into anxiety using what you now know. If you feel it very physically, use that as a warning signal. If your thoughts act as the giveaway, start observing critical mind-jabs. Noticing where it affects you first will give you options for interrupting anxiety loops and creating more positive mind maps.

What Makes You Feel Anxious?

The next six pages are dedicated to helping you identify the external things that make you feel anxious.

What social events or responsibilities do you dread?

What professional responsibilities make you tense before they've even begun?

What particular settings or types of places do you find yourself avoiding?

Are there specific types of people you'd rather not be around?

Which aspects of your routine make you most tense?

When you cancel or procrastinate, what event, chore, or obligation are you avoiding?

The Build-Up

Sometimes long-term anxieties can affect how you respond to short-term or everyday annoyances. Starting at the "eruption point," work your way down to the deeper layers.

Eruption point: What recent, relatively small event(s) tipped you over the edge, causing you to lash out or shut down?

Upper layer: Write some routine annoyances that can feel part of a larger pattern, such as being late, plans being changed or canceled, or receiving criticism.

Medium layer: Here, list situational stressors. The kind that don't last forever, but feel overwhelming at the time, such as a breakup, moving, or losing your job.

Bottom layer: Note down any constant long-term anxieties, such as financial instability, family conflict, or health concerns.

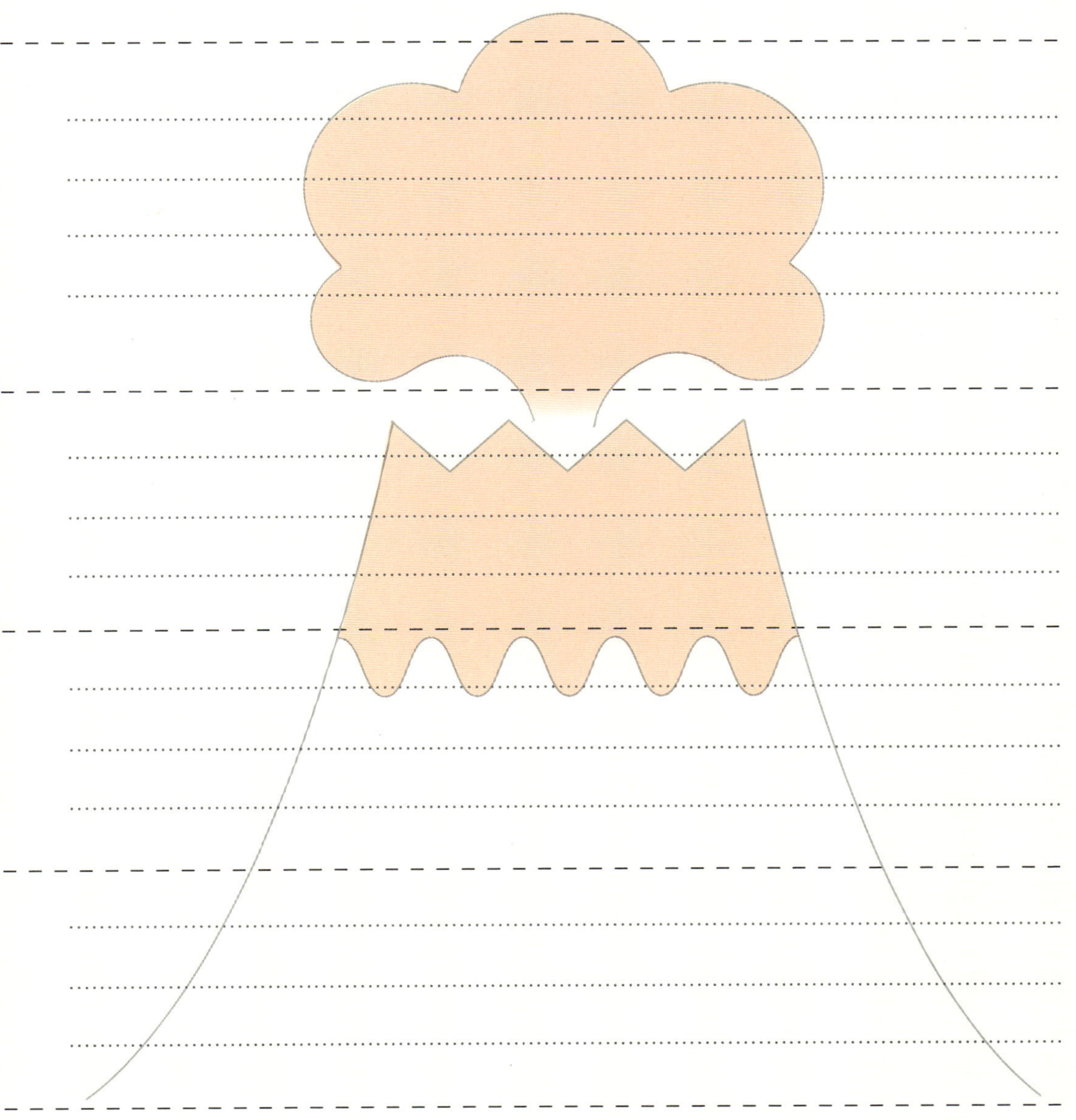

How might your eruption points (see previous pages) have been impacted by deeper, longer-term anxieties?

What did this teach you about your stress threshold?

What do you notice first when you respond to eruption points—your mood, body, behavior, or thoughts?

What do you notice first with more longer-term anxieties—your mood, body, behavior, or thoughts?

How might you use this knowledge going forward?

You can't stop anxiety, but you can change how you respond to it.

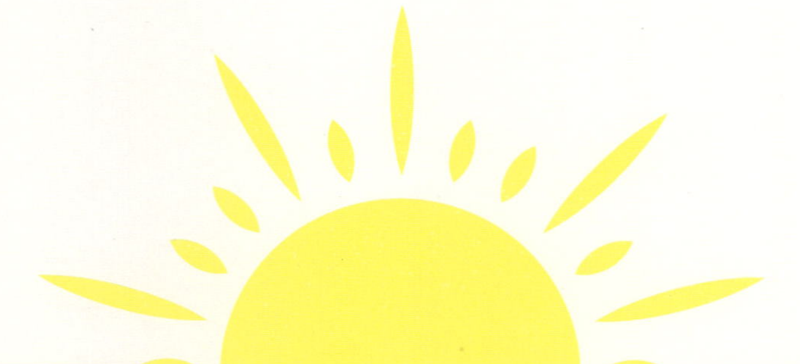

Notes to Self

Repeating affirmations to yourself can help to calm both body and mind when you're spiraling. Fill in the blank spaces with true and positive statements that are personal to you.

This feeling is temporary. I will get through it.

I can do hard things even when I feel anxious.

I don't need to have all the answers right now.

My anxiety does not define me.

Thoughts aren't facts.

Thoughts Aren't Facts

How often do you trust your thoughts to be 100% true?

○ Always ○ Mostly ○ Sometimes ○ Not often (I usually question my thoughts)

How does your mood affect the things you tell yourself?

How does your environment—where you are, what you're doing, and who you're with, as well as your health—affect what you tell yourself?

What kinds of thoughts feel most "true" in the moment but then tend not to hold up later?

What would surprise people if they heard you speak your thoughts out loud?

Imagine you could observe your thoughts objectively without automatically believing them. How would you feel?

Fact-Check Your Thoughts

Write down some recent thoughts you stated to yourself as facts, and work through the questions below.

Thought	Mood	Was this fact, fear, or opinion?
Example: "My friends didn't invite me to a group event because they're mad at me."	Rejected, hurt, vulnerable	Fear

Thoughts are just opinions put forward by your biased brain.

What's another possibility that could be true?	What would you tell a friend thinking this?
They thought I was busy or that someone else had invited me.	"Ask why you weren't invited. Don't assume—find out the facts and go from there."

Reflect

Can you identify a belief you hold about yourself that's not helpful and not true?

When experiencing a strong emotion, do you find it easiest to tune into your moods, body, behavior, or thoughts first—and how can you use that knowledge going forward?

How has learning about your anxiety made you feel more confident about being able to manage it?

How do you feel about your anxiety now?

How do you rate your ability to cope with your anxiety now on a scale of 1 to 10?

○ 1 ○ 2 ○ 3 ○ 4 ○ 5 ○ 6 ○ 7 ○ 8 ○ 9 ○ 10

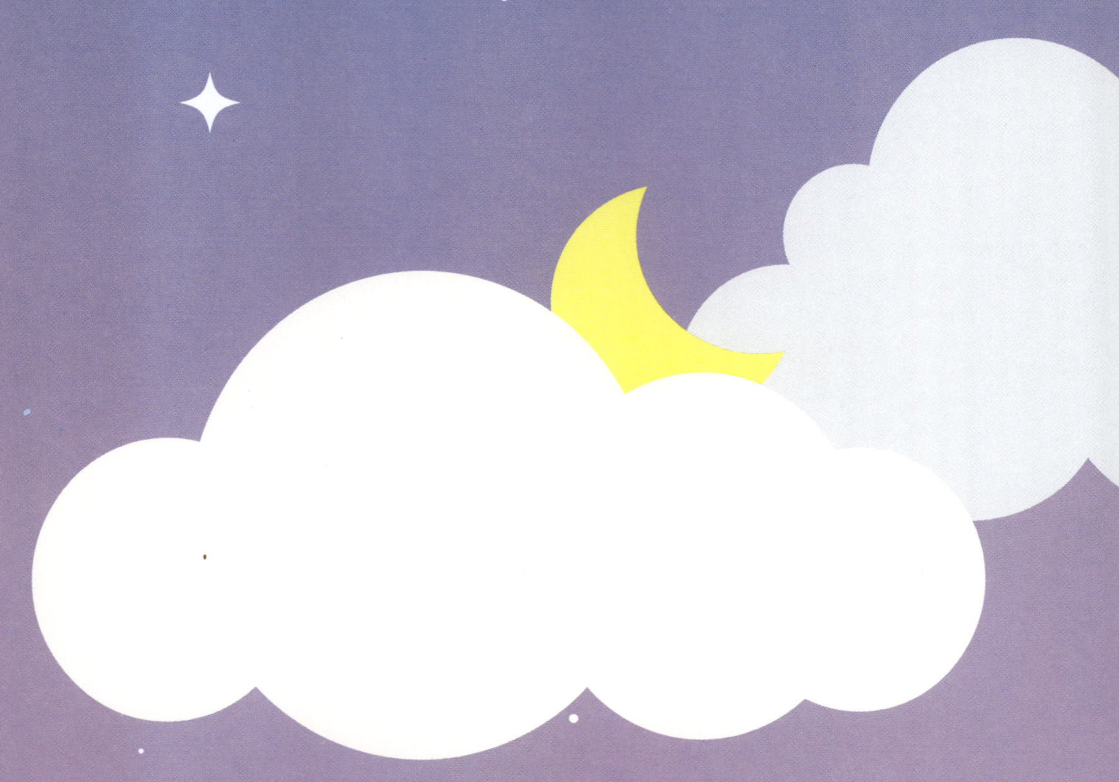

PART TWO

Body Talk

Anxiety can make you feel awful physically. Yet, you can use the discomfort as an early-warning system, interrupting negative cycles before they spiral. Here you'll learn how to spot the signs so you can calm your body and therefore also your mind.

Listening to Your Body

What happens in your body when you start to feel anxious?

Do you always recognize these signs, or do you sometimes mistake them for other physical states, such as sickness or caffeine overload?

How long can symptoms last before you notice them?

How do these physical feelings affect your thoughts and behavior?

Do you associate any other moods with these feelings in your body, aside from anxiety?

What's a common situation that makes you feel physically anxious?

How about one that makes you feel physically calm?

Map the Tension

On the figure on the left, shade in areas where you feel anxiety in your body. On the figure on the right, use different colors, press harder, or crosshatch to map how long each feeling tends to last.

Where you feel it

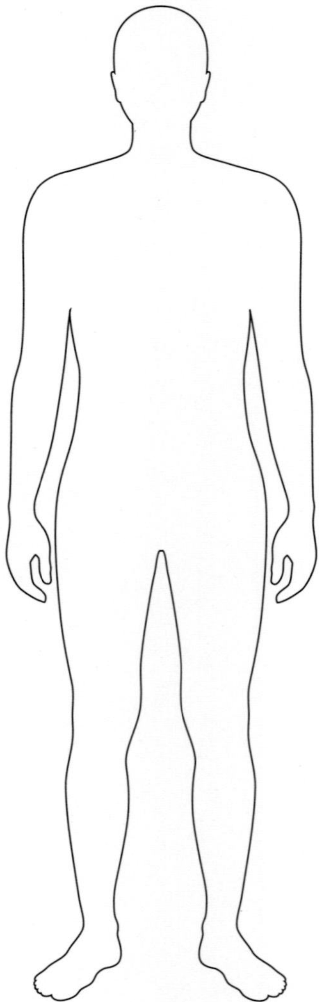

How long it lasts

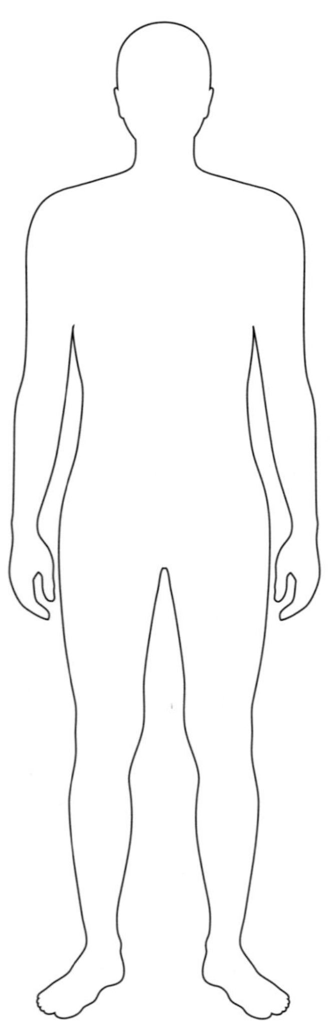

Ground Yourself

When you're feeling anxious, try this mindfulness exercise. By concentrating on your senses, you can pull your focus to the present to help calm both body and mind. It can be done anywhere and anytime. Swap senses for emotions if needed. For example, if you can't taste anything, change this for "name all the emotions that you feel."

5: Name **five** things you can see.

....

....

4: Touch **four** different textures.

....

....

3: Listen out for **three** specific sounds.

....

....

2: Differentiate between **two** distinct smells.

....

....

1: Identify **one** flavor you can taste.

....

....

The Three Fs: Fight, Flight, or Freeze

Fight:
Confront or attack the "threat"

Flight:
Run away from the "threat"

Freeze:
Assess the danger or "play dead"

What are they?

Instant, automatic responses to perceived danger where your body either "fights," "flees," or "freezes." Adrenaline surges, causing a racing heartbeat, rapid breathing, muscle tension, heightened alertness, and sometimes numbness or immobility.

How does it feel?

You might feel tingly, sweaty, nauseous, and experience rapid or shallow breathing, tunnel vision, trembling, and dry mouth.

What's the problem?

The Three Fs can't differentiate between genuine danger and everyday stress, preparing you in exactly the same way for both. The good news? You can learn how to manage these reactions.

When experiencing the symptoms of fight or flight, do you tend to respond by confronting the situation (fight) or by distancing yourself from it (flight)?

When have you previously frozen in a stressful moment?

What kinds of situations tend to trigger fight, flight, or freeze for you?

How long does the feeling last, and what helps to calm your body down?

When have you experienced "fawn" (sometimes described as the "fourth F")—people pleasing to defuse tension?

Set a timer for ten minutes and use this space to free-write whatever is on your mind, perhaps related to The Three Fs.

Mind Map

Work through a recent time you experienced fight or flight. You can leave the event box blank if the response happened because of worrying thoughts, strong emotions, or something you did (behavior). Freeze can be challenging to map as your body essentially goes "offline," impairing memory.

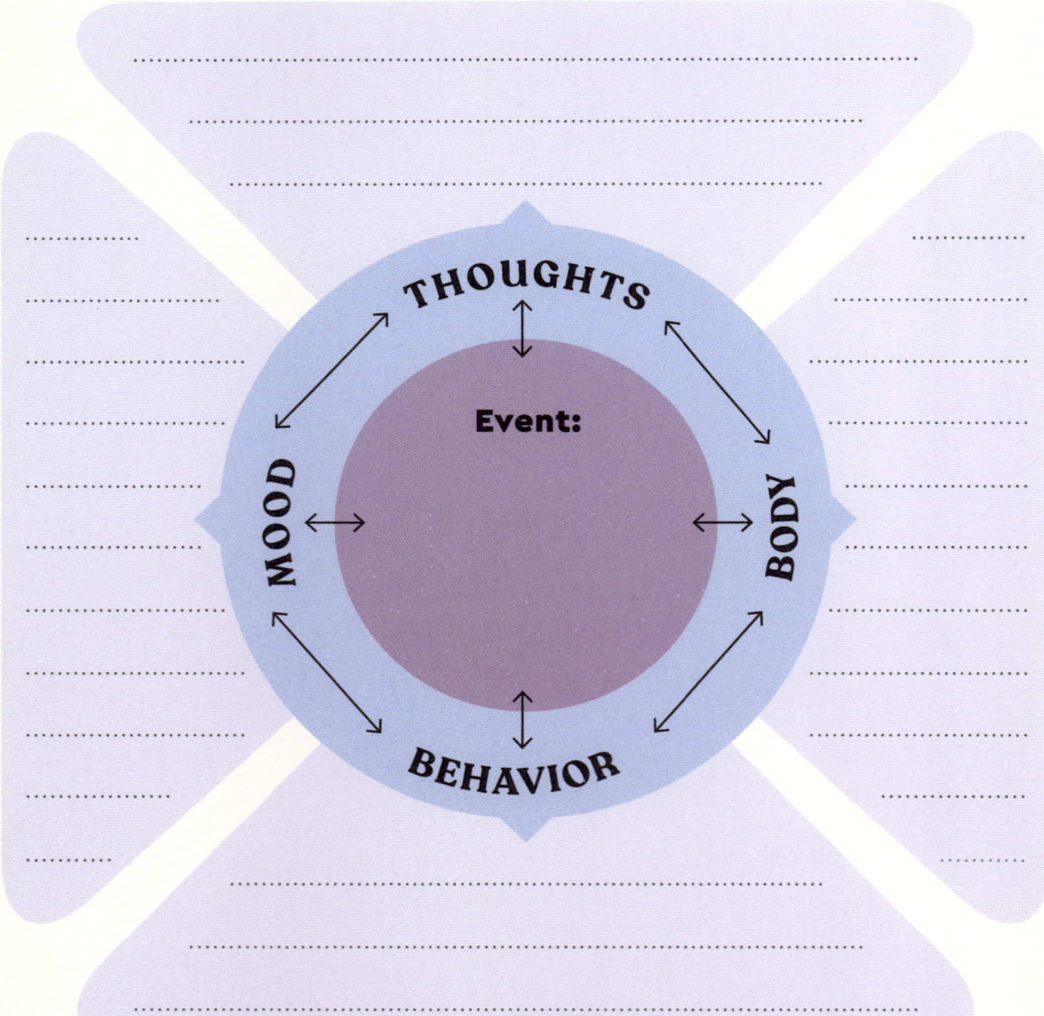

Anti-Anxiety Loop

Fill in this anti-anxiety loop using a time you calmed yourself down from fight or flight. Maybe you challenged a thought, soothed your body, or altered your behavior. How did that impact your mood?

BEHAVIOR

THOUGHTS

BODY

MOOD

Which of the Three Fs do you notice in people close to you, and how do you usually respond to them?

How does it help knowing your body is simply trying to protect you?

What personal Three F patterns have you begun to recognize?

A Maze Moment

Finding a path to your calm? It might take some false starts, but trust in the journey. This grounding exercise will pull your mind to the present, interrupting anxiety loops. Remember to breathe deeply and mindfully as you go.

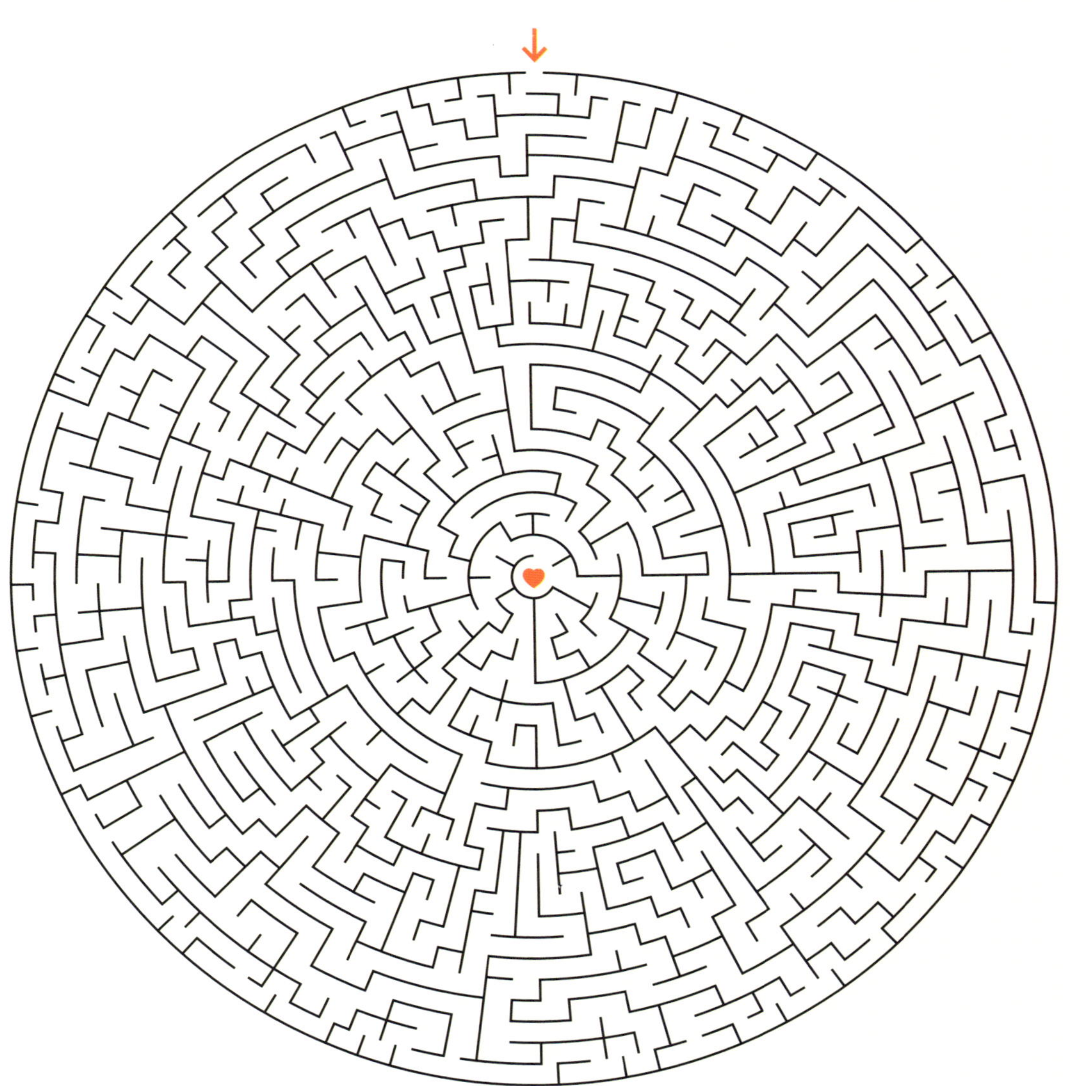

In This Moment, I am Safe

Work through these questions to ground yourself in the present, observe and ease physical symptoms, and build a sense of trust in your body.

What physical sensations do you notice right now?

Check the most appropriate words below (if any) to help describe your physical sensations:

- ○ Loose
- ○ Relaxed
- ○ Light
- ○ Warm
- ○ Tight
- ○ Stiff
- ○ Heavy
- ○ Cold

What does feeling physically calm mean to you?

What small actions might bring comfort to your body right now? (For example, placing a hand on your chest, stretching, rhythmic patting, or deep breathing.)

....

....

....

....

What proof do you have that you are safe in this moment?

....

....

....

....

....

How might you recreate that feeling elsewhere?

....

....

....

....

Repeat the phrase, "In this moment, I am safe" five times to yourself and really focus on it. How does your body respond?

....

....

....

....

Learn Your Body Language

What does anxiety look like for you?

Posture and body language	Speech
◯ Hunched ◯ Slouching ◯ Tense or stiff ◯ Swaying ◯ Fidgeting ◯ Avoiding eye contact ◯ Crossed arms ◯ Trying to make yourself smaller	◯ Rushed ◯ Apologetic ◯ Defensive ◯ Self-correcting ◯ Mumbling ◯ Over-explaining ◯ Laughing or giggling for no reason
Appearance	**Actions**
◯ Unkempt ◯ Nondescript clothes ◯ Uncomfortable ◯ Unclean ◯ Compulsively clean or groomed ◯ Overdressed ◯ Underdressed	◯ Walking timidly or pacing ◯ Avoiding or procrastinating ◯ Making repetitive movements ◯ People pleasing (fawning) ◯ Self-sabotaging ◯ Aggressive gestures ◯ Canceling plans ◯ Overcompensating

For one week, any time you find yourself looking or acting anxious, intentionally do the opposite—act and look calm. Track what happens in this table.

What were you doing?	What did you change?	How did it make you feel?
Example: Standing at the edge of a group with arms folded.	I uncrossed my arms, stood tall, and contributed to the chat.	More confident. Everyone was really nice to me.

What does calm or in control look like for you?

....

....

....

....

How did acting calm affect how you actually felt?

....

....

....

....

Visualize Calm

Visualization is a tried and tested technique for finding calm. Through practice, you can escape to a getaway you've created in your mind, transporting yourself there whenever things get tough.

Go somewhere you won't be disturbed, get comfortable, take several long deep breaths, release any tension in your body…and get ready to escape.

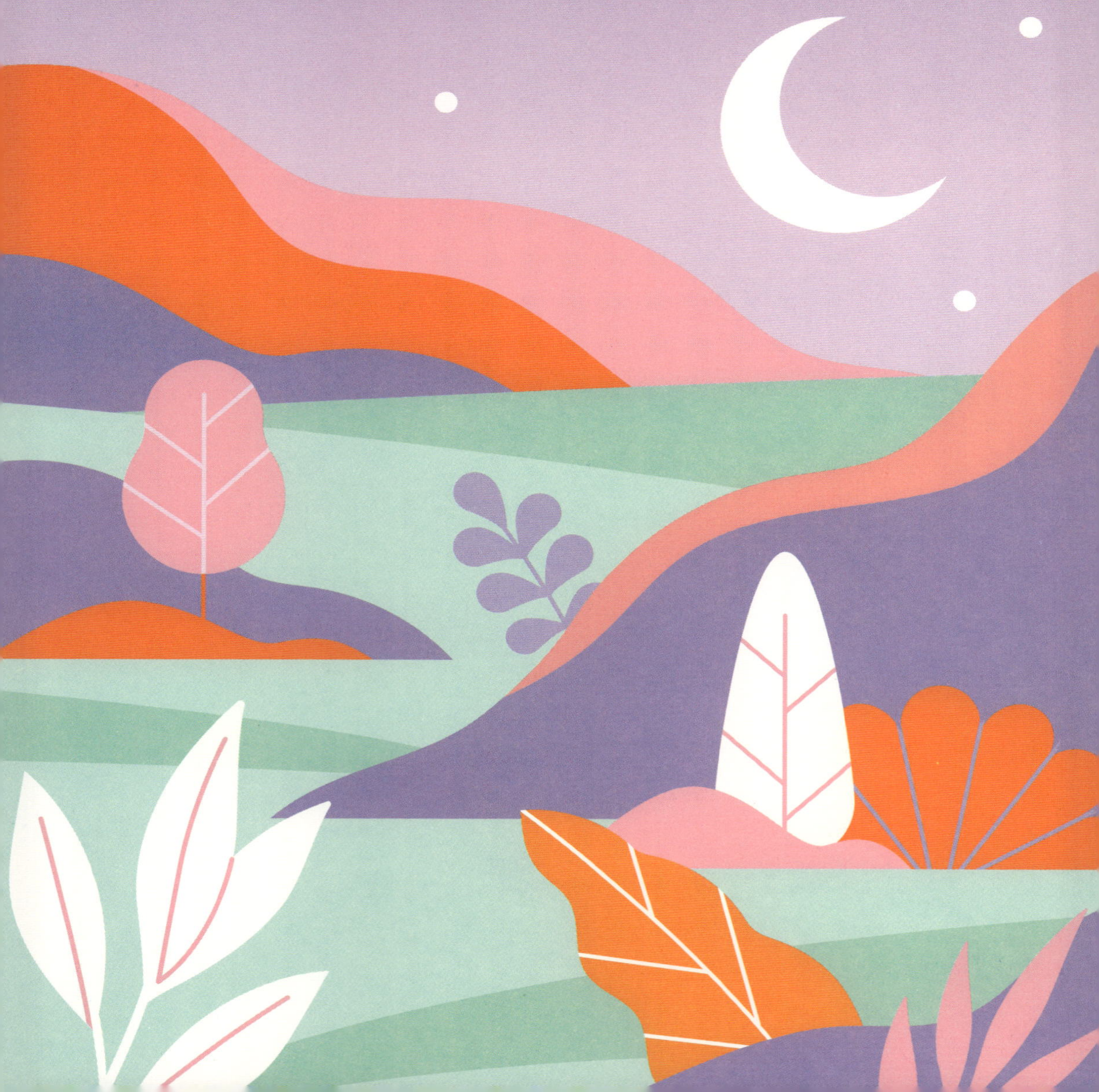

Imagine a scene where you can feel absolutely at peace, such as a beach, a forest, or a secret cabin. Where are you?

How do you get to this place? For example, do you follow a path, arrive by boat, open a door, or walk down some stairs?

What do you do there? Is there a cool mountain stream to dip your toes in or maybe a roaring fire to cozy up beside?

Describe everything around you. What's above, below, and beside you. What can you see, hear, smell, taste, and touch?

How do you feel emotionally and physically?

How do you know when you're ready to leave—and how does the scene then end?

Your Getaway Scrapbook

Use this page as a scrapbook for getaway ideas. Fill it with images of calming inspiration, like a visualization mood board. Or, use the space for a free-writing exercise, describing your getaway in detail.

Stress Tracker

	Day 1	Day 2	Day 3
What happened and where were you?			
What were you doing and who was there?			
How did your body respond?			
What thoughts did you notice?			
What emotions did you notice?			
What actions did you take?			
How anxious were you? (rate 1-10)			

For seven days, list anything that makes you feel stressed, whether big or small, and answer the questions that follow. This will help you to see patterns, giving you opportunities to make changes later on. This is also a useful way to work out what doesn't stress you out. Maybe you actually enjoy doing the laundry or dropping off mail because they offer quiet moments.

Day 4	Day 5	Day 6	Day 7

Healthy Habits

What healthy and helpful habits would you like to start or continue? They don't have to be only about physical health, but life in general! For example, maybe you want to exercise more, read more books, put in regular calls with your friends, or prioritize sleep.

Healthy habits to start or continue	How will you hold yourself accountable?	Did you do it?
		○
		○
		○
		○
		○
		○
		○
		○

What unhealthy or unhelpful habits would you like to try to stop? For example, maybe you'd like to cut down on caffeine or alcohol, stop doomscrolling, or limit your social media use. Use your body as a guide. How do you feel physically during and afterward?

Unhealthy habits to stop	How will you hold yourself accountable?	Did you stop?
		○
		○
		○
		○
		○
		○
		○
		○

Reflect

Were there any physical responses you hadn't connected to anxiety before?

In what ways do you feel more aware of how your mind is connected to your body, and vice versa?

How can you use your body as a warning system for when anxiety is creeping up on you?

What tools help to calm your body down?

How do you rate your ability to cope with your anxiety now on a scale of 1 to 10?

○ 1 ○ 2 ○ 3 ○ 4 ○ 5 ○ 6 ○ 7 ○ 8 ○ 9 ○ 10

PART THREE

Mind Over Matter

Are you ready to meet your inner critic? Fair warning: they might speak nonsense, but they are somehow still convincing. Learn how to spot anxious thoughts and worries so you can choose whether to act on them, challenge them, ignore them, laugh at them, or simply let them go.

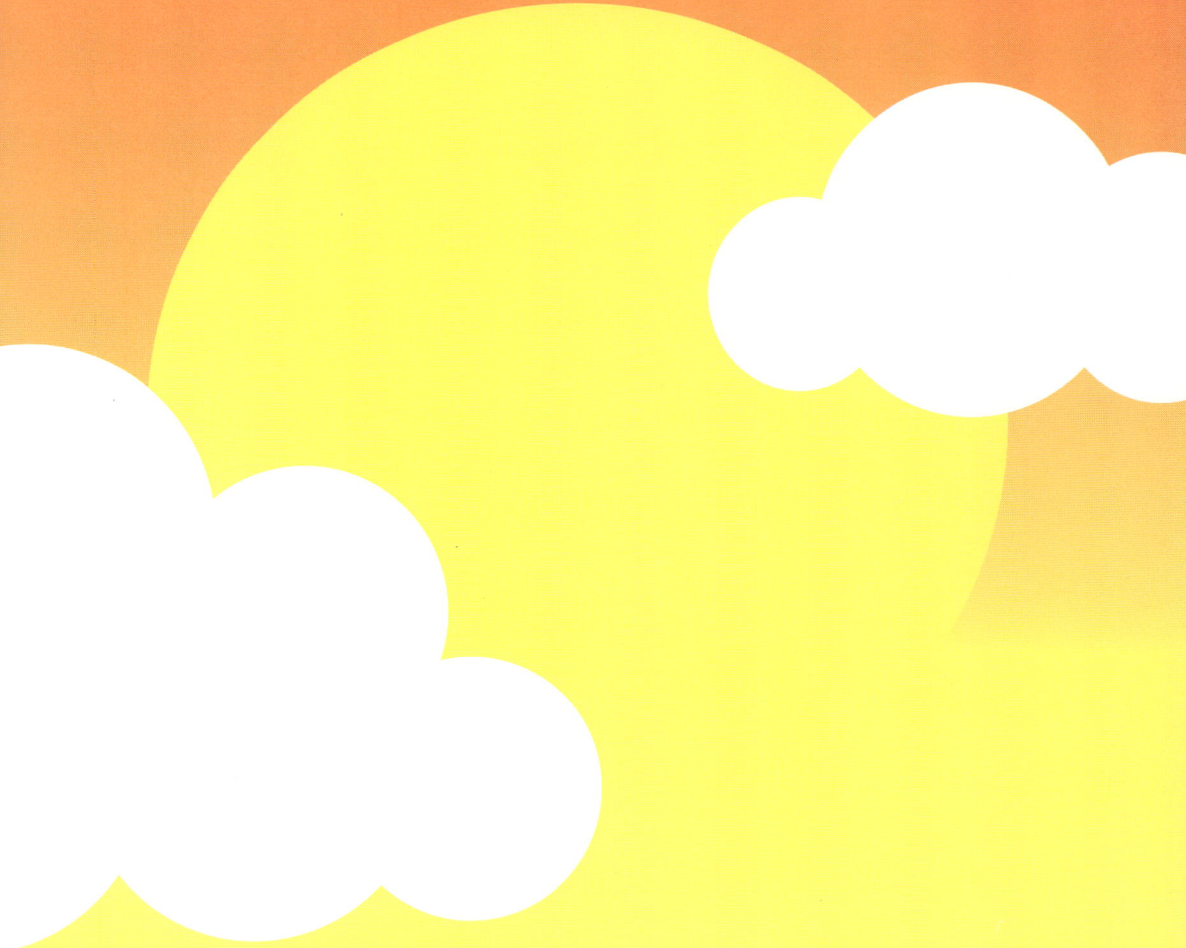

Give Your Thoughts Space

What thoughts have been looping through your mind recently?

Are they mostly thoughts masquerading as facts (statements), self-criticism, or worries (concerns about the future)?

Do you often challenge them, or do you tend to let them guide you?

Is there one thought you try not to think about?

Is it about something within your control?

What do your anxious thoughts assume about you and the world?

Meet Your Inner Critic

Your inner critic is the voice in your head spouting so-called "facts." These are only biased opinions, yet they'll inevitably make you feel bad about yourself. They come in many forms.

Catastrophizing: Overestimating the danger and underestimating your ability to cope. List three catastrophizing thoughts that have affected you in the past.

Disqualifying the positive: Explaining away or ignoring compliments, positive feedback, or good luck. When did you last play down a positive comment, compliment, or something that went your way?

Magical thinking: Believing your thoughts can influence outcomes. (Not so!) Think of a time when you used negative magical thinking. What about a positive example?

Mind reading: Creating narratives around what you believe other people are thinking and acting accordingly. When did you recently act on a belief based on mind reading?

Always and never: Negative things "always" happen while positive things "never" happen. (There's also black-and-white thinking, where things are either right or wrong, good or bad, with no gray area.) Think of one example of "always and never" thinking and one of "black and white" thinking.

Fortune telling: You dust off your crystal ball and predict negative future outcomes. When is the last time you predicted you'd come up short?

Mind Map

Choose an example of a recent self-critical thought and mind map your inner critic below. How did it affect your body, behavior, and mood? Can you see places where you could stop this cycle? (Leave the event box blank if the thought came from nowhere.)

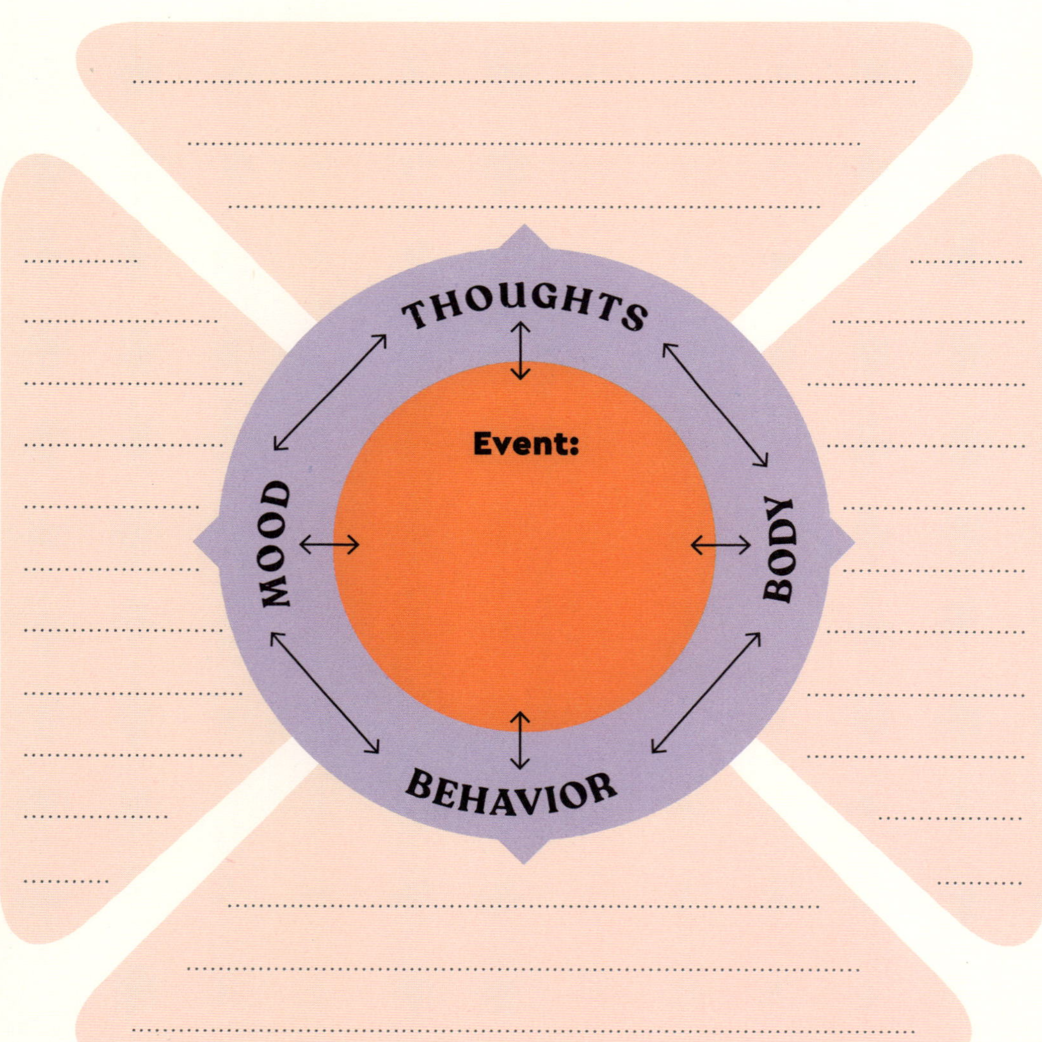

Which type of negative thoughts do you experience the most, and why do you think that might be?

Are most of your negative thoughts focused on one subject, such as work, friends, or comparisons?

Ask yourself these questions when you next catch a self-critical thought:

1. What type of negative thought is this?
2. How strongly do I believe it, on a scale of 1 to 10, with 10 being full belief?
3. What evidence contradicts it?
4. What would a fairer view be?
5. What would I tell a friend who thought this way?
6. How strongly do I believe the negative thought now, on the same scale from 1 to 10?

Bravery Badges

Everyone deserves achievement badges! Award yourself one of the below badges the next time you're courageous.

Negative Thought Slayer

☐ I overcame this negative thought:

____
____
____

☐ Bravery score (1-5)

Reality Checker

☐ I challenged this self-doubt:

____
____
____

☐ Bravery score (1-5)

Fear Facer

☐ I did this thing that scared me:

____
____
____

☐ Bravery score (1-5)

Action Taker

☐ I took control of this situation:

____
____
____

☐ Bravery score (1-5)

Grace Giver

☐ I cut myself some slack when:

____
____
____

☐ Bravery score (1-5)

This is about how **you** felt, not how you think other people would judge what you did.

The Compliment Cache

When you feel low, it's easy to dismiss compliments. This tracker helps give them the attention they deserve. Log at least three examples of positive feedback you get this week, no matter how small.

Compliment	**1**	**2**	**3**
What was the situation?			
How did the compliment make you feel emotionally?			
What happened within your body?			
What are you most proud of about it?			
If you simply accepted the praise, without dismissing it publicly or personally, how would you feel?			

Thinking Traps

Negative thoughts can catch you in recurring thinking traps that are tough to escape, leading to anxiety loops. These prompts will help you to recognize when you might be about to trip into a trap.

How do you usually respond to criticism or disapproval?

When was the last time you gave someone else praise or a compliment? Does that come easily to you?

Do you celebrate other people's successes or see them as a reflection of what you're not doing?

Do you ever reflect criticism you hear about others on to yourself, and then worry about it?

How often do you behave defensively in the expectation of receiving bad news or criticism?

Tip: Ask yourself, "Is this thought helpful right now?" If yes, what action can it help you to take? If no, say, "Thanks, mind, I hear you," and move on.

The Likely Pie

1. Choose one negative thought that's bothering you.
2. List all possible outcomes, from best-case scenario to end-of-the-world bad.
3. Imagine your worry as a pie. Divide it into slices by giving a percentage to each outcome based on how likely it is. If you're unsure, ask yourself how a friend would judge it.

Example: Event: I made a fool of myself at a work party.

Possible outcomes (from best to worst):

A: No one noticed at all.

B: A few people noticed and laughed it off.

C: My boss mentions it, but in a jokey way.

D: My boss flags it up as a mild warning.

E: I am severely disciplined.

F: I lose my job and never work again.

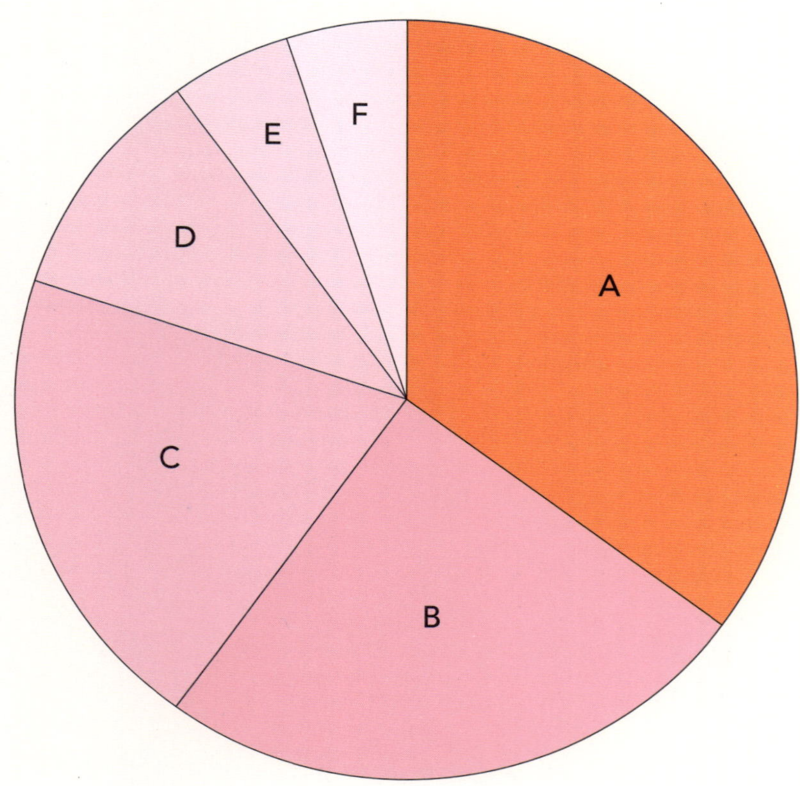

Event: ______________________________

Possible outcomes (from best to worst):

A: ______________________________

B: ______________________________

C: ______________________________

D: ______________________________

E: ______________________________

F: ______________________________

The Second Arrow

The Second Arrow is a mindfulness concept that explains how we sometimes inflict unnecessary pain on ourselves—and how we can choose not to.

THE SECOND ARROW

The second arrow: Responding with self-criticism, self-doubt, rumination, anger, worry, guilt, shame, or comparing yourself to others.

THE FIRST ARROW

The first arrow: An emotionally painful experience.

While we may not be able to avoid the first arrow, we can absolutely avoid shooting ourselves with a second.

Catching the Second Arrow

Before firing that second arrow, pause and ask yourself if you really want to pile on unnecessary hurt. You have agency here. You can choose.

First arrow: The facts

1. What do you know for a fact happened?
2. What emotions did you notice?
3. What happened in your body?
4. What did you immediately do?

Loading the second arrow: The story

1. What story did you tell yourself about the first arrow?
2. What fortune telling, catastrophizing, or mind-reading took place?
3. How did that affect your mood, body, and behavior?
4. What are you telling yourself you "should" or "shouldn't" have done?

The pause

1. Is this second arrow (this story you're telling) helpful?
2. Does it make you feel better or worse?
3. How does it make you want to act?
4. Does it make you feel more or less in control?

Returning the second arrow to its quiver

How can you respond to just the first arrow?

From Catastrophe to Calm

Fill in this tracker to gain perspective on worst-case scenarios, helping you feel more in control.

Catastrophe

What happened or is happening?

→

Worst-case scenario fear

↓

What are the facts?

←

Possible solution (1)

↓

Possible solution (2)

→

Possible solution (3)

↓

Possible solution (4)

....

....

....

Which solution(s) will best help your anxiety and solve the problem?

....

....

Break the plan down into steps

....

....

....

....

....

....

....

....

How and when will you start?

....

....

....

How did it go?

....

....

....

Do you feel better for having done something, even if it didn't work out? Y/N

....

What next?

1. Start the process again based on a new situation.
2. Try a different solution.
3. No new steps needed, it's sorted!

The Control Center

Here you'll learn about the three types of worry and how much control you really have over future outcomes.

What ifs
These are worries about hypothetical problems that don't exist yet and probably never will. When they spiral, your body and mood react as if they're real, impacting your behavior.

Worries you DO have control over
These concerns are real. You can exert some control over them by making proactive plans or taking action.

Worries you DON'T have control over
These concerns are also real, but you can't do anything about them. These are things like aging, the weather, and accidents.

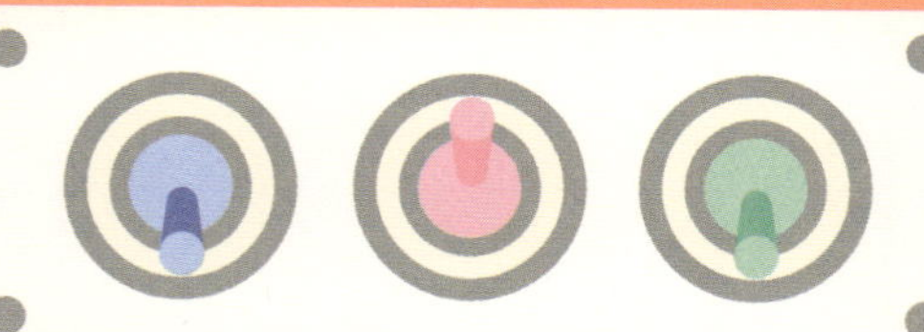

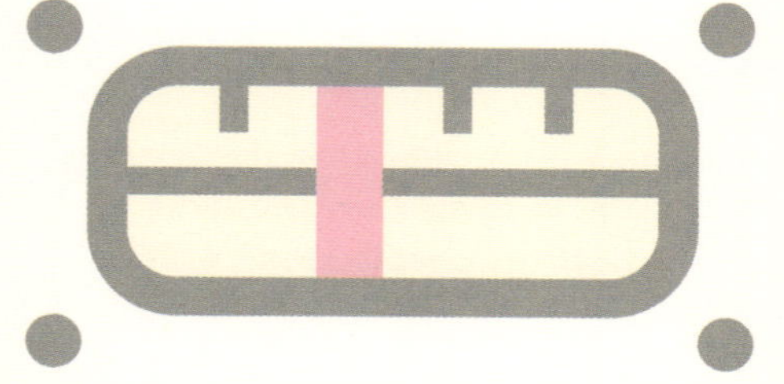

Banishing "What Ifs"

What are some common "what if..." thoughts you have?

When do they happen most: What time of day, what mood are you in, how are you feeling physically, and what are you doing?

Roughly how many of your past biggest "what ifs" never happened?

What Is Your Worry?

Pick three worries and follow your way through this worry control center.

Is this worry real?

NO, it's hypothetical

Can you do anything about it?

NO

Let the worry go

- Practice grounding techniques **(see pages 43 and 174)**.
- Distract yourself through exercise or doing something creative.
- Try visualization **(see pages 56 to 59)**.
- Try the "so what?" technique: Follow your worry to its natural conclusion and then say, "So what?" It can help keep things in perspective.

1.

2.

3.

YES, it's real

YES

Make a plan

- Break down the worry into smaller, more manageable steps.
- Make realistic and timely plans for how you will face each step.
- Ask your friends or family for help if you're struggling.
- Don't have time to make a plan now? Schedule it in your calendar!

What has surprised you most about learning how, when, and why you worry?

Do you see worrying as a form of caring? If so, what are some more positive and proactive ways of showing you care?

What's a recent situation that went well despite you NOT worrying about it? Does this make you think differently about worrying being helpful?

Fill in these circles with a recent snowballing "What if." Start with the worst-case worry and work backward to the original worry, which was likely a much smaller concern.

Start Here

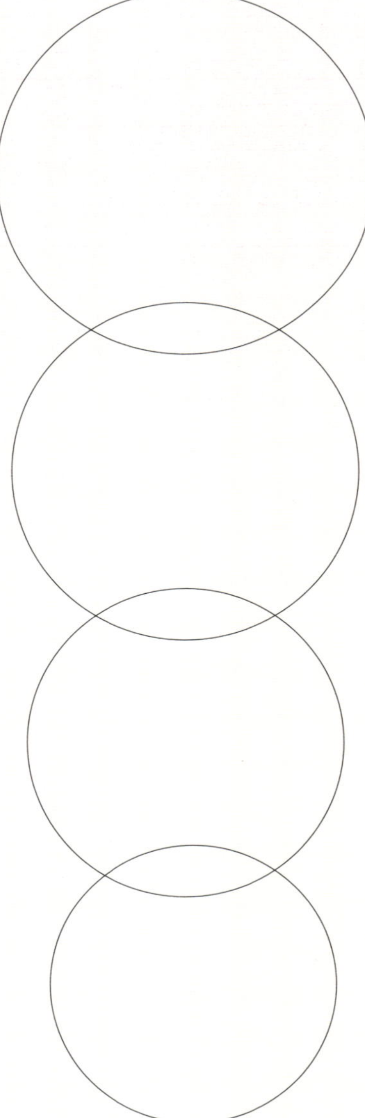

Self-fulfilling Prophecies

A self-fulfilling prophecy is when your expectations—either positive or negative—influence your behavior in ways that cause those expectations to come true.

Describe a recent time you predicted something would go wrong and behaved as if that thought was true.

If the outcome was indeed bad, how much do you think your prophecy and resulting behavior played a part?

If the outcome was good, what reason did you attribute to it?

Have assumptions about how others see you affected how you behave?

What kind of satisfaction do you get at being proved "right" in these scenarios?

Mind Map

This mind map is about a positive self-fulfilling prophecy. Start with an event you felt really confident would turn out well—that did end up having a great outcome!—and work through from there.

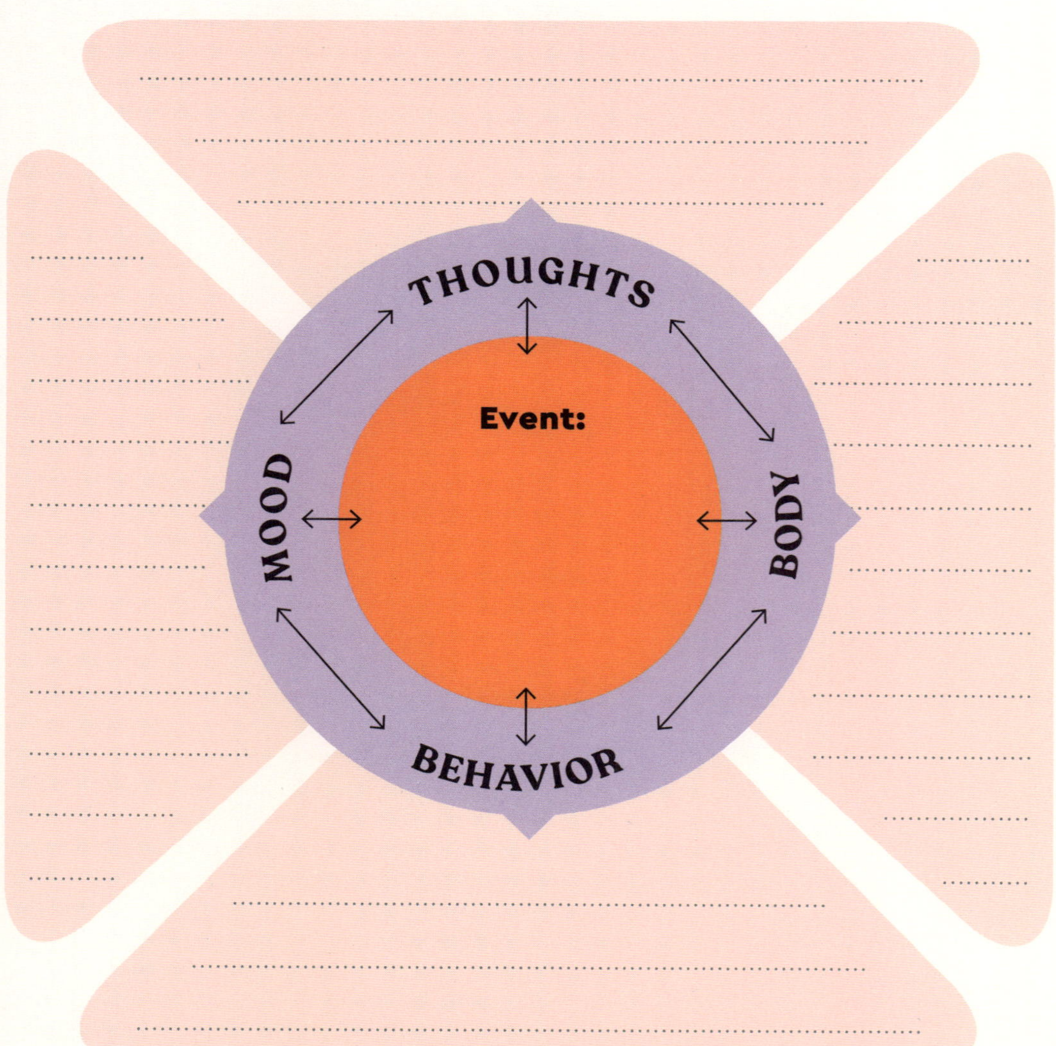

Anti-Anxiety Loop

Fill in this anti-anxiety loop starting with a thought about a recent success you enjoyed, paying attention to the knock-on effect of each section.

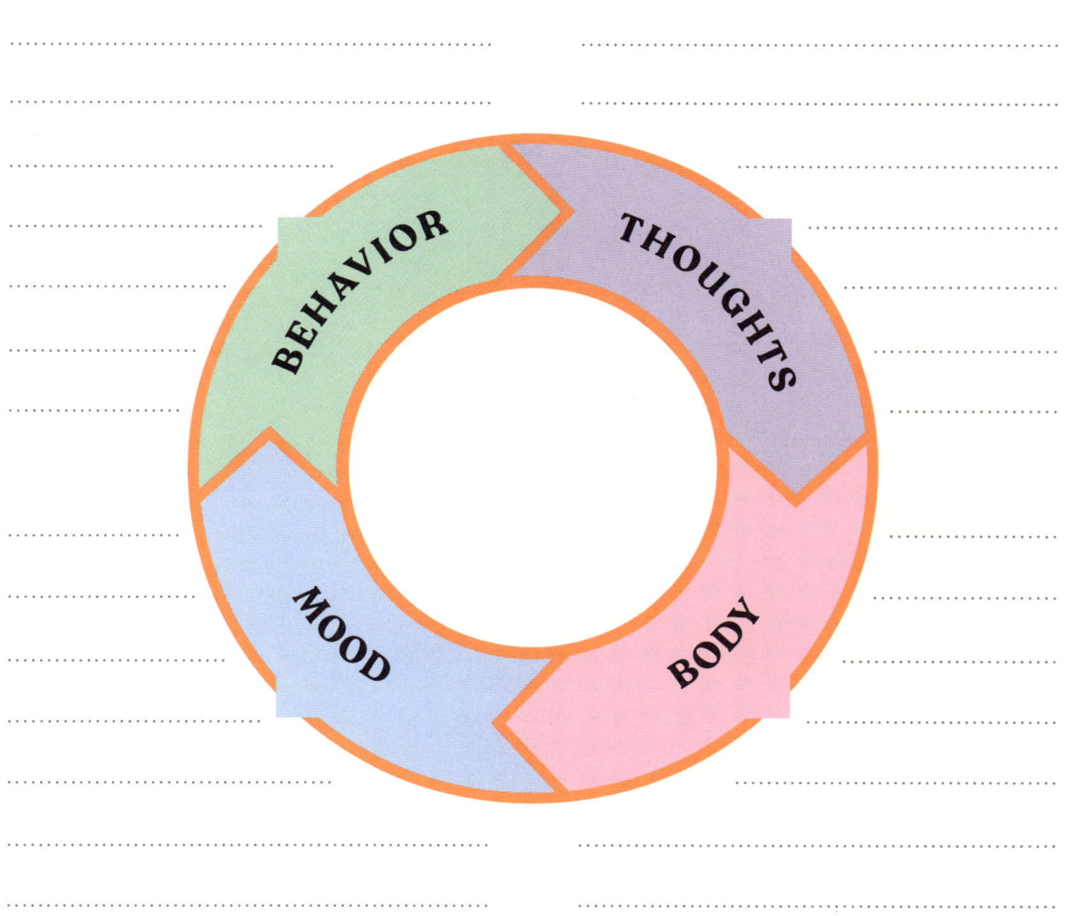

Designated Doubt Time

Scheduling time to worry might sound unusual, but it can help put things in perspective. Each day, set aside 15 minutes to dwell on doubts. Every time a worry pops up during the day, tell yourself, "I'll think about it during my designated doubt time," and move on. Then, during your doubt time, answer these questions.

What is worrying you?

....

....

....

....

....

How do you feel seeing these worries listed out?

....

....

....

....

Which category of worry are they? Are they hypothetical "what ifs," concerns within your control, or concerns out of your control?

....

....

....

....

....

Set an additional 10-minute timer and use this space for free-journaling. Write down any thoughts you have about your worries and how you find scheduling doubt time.

Reflect

How has your understanding of how you experience anxious thoughts changed?

What did you find most challenging about completing this section?

What habits do you want to develop based on what you've learned?

How might letting anxious thoughts go or challenging them affect your daily life?

How do you feel about your thoughts and how they've impacted you now?

Going forward, how much will you allow your thoughts to dictate what you do, without pausing to question them first?

How do you rate your ability to cope with your anxiety now on a scale of 1 to 10?

○ 1 ○ 2 ○ 3 ○ 4 ○ 5 ○ 6 ○ 7 ○ 8 ○ 9 ○ 10

PART FOUR

Best Behavior

You may have noticed that your anxiety can lead to self-defeating behaviors. Part Four will help you identify which actions are serving you well and which most definitely aren't.

Unpacking Anxiety Acts

What are your go-to behaviors when you feel anxious?

Do you tend to do more or do less when you're feeling on edge?

How does anxiety change the way you speak or act around others?

What do you procrastinate over or avoid completely?

What do you redo over and over again because it's not "perfect"?

What behaviors help you feel calm?

Stop Ghosting Your To-Do List

Avoidance and procrastination are incredibly common anxiety behaviors because they seem to offer short-term relief. But this is always at the cost of long-term angst. Work through these prompts to discover how these behaviors affect how you handle challenges.

What tasks are you procrastinating (postponing) or avoiding (ghosting) right now and why?

What does your procrastination or avoidance look like?

Does it usually work? Do you usually think less about your task, or more?

How does avoidance and procrastination make you feel emotionally and physically?

Do you mostly feel overwhelmed by external demands (what's being asked of you) or internal demands (what you're asking of yourself)?

How much time, energy, and headspace does postponing or ghosting take up?

Would knowing exactly what you're facing feel better or worse than tackling a big unknown?

Face Your To-Do List

Break any big tasks on your to-do list down into smaller steps and give each smaller task a time slot so you can see an end point.

Which tasks can you delegate or outsource? Let some stuff go!

Which tasks can you get rid of completely?

How will you protect your time in the future? Could you turn some things down or be more honest about when you can deliver something?

You Can Do It

Fill in this tracker with tasks you're facing or have already faced. You might be surprised to find it proves that the actual outcomes are very different from what you feared might happen.

Continuously dodging an issue means that you never disprove your anxious thoughts, which then adds more angst on top. Facing things, no matter how scary, will make you feel immediately calmer because you're taking action.

What are/were you avoiding?	What do/did you fear happening?	How anxious do/did you feel (1-10)?	What happened after facing it?

Swap Self-Sabotage for Self-Trust

We can get in our own way when we feel anxious. Answer these prompts to dig into why and how you might trip yourself up.

Note down a recent time you deliberately sabotaged something you were doing.

What made you behave that way? Was it a fear of failure, fear of change, imposter syndrome, overwhelm, need for control, or something else?

What stories did you tell yourself to justify doing it?

How did you feel emotionally and physically after you had self-sabotaged?

When did you last succeed at something you were scared could go wrong?

List at least four reasons that you DO deserve good things.

Permission Not to Be Perfect

We strive to be perfect in areas of life where we're most scared of feeling vulnerable, rejected, ridiculed, or judged. The following pages will help you to identify and challenge unrealistic expectations.

What does "perfect" mean to you, right now?

When do you put the most pressure on yourself not to make mistakes or show flaws?

What are you afraid will happen if something isn't as good as it could have been?

Where did this drive come from and what aggravates it? (For example, from social media, family, friends, or where you live.)

Do you find "perfect" people or those who show flaws more approachable, and why?

How do you think your need for things to be just right affects others?

That's Just Perfect

You can successfully challenge perfectionism and rethink "failure." For one month, check a box any time you let go of unrealistic standards. Try to check each box a few times!

- **You ask yourself, "What did I learn from this?"**
- **You deliberately do something you're bad at.**
- **You laugh at yourself.**
- **You celebrate trying rather than succeeding.**
- **You let go of an unhelpful standard.**
- **You choose rest over improvement.**
- **You recognize that things aren't always black and white, but often gray.**

You haven't failed. You're just taking the scenic route to success.

Self-Worth, Not Scoreboards

Comparing is human nature. Where it gets tricky is when you only ever compare your worst bits to other people's best bits.

When did you last compare yourself to someone?

What areas of life do you tend to compare most?

Do you compare yourself mostly to people online or in real life? Why?

How do you usually feel after these comparisons: motivated, inspired, and proud, or anxious, sad, and despondent?

What assumptions are you making about the people you're comparing yourself to?

What steps can you take to make fairer comparisons—fairer to you and others?

Being Mode

"Being mode" is the opposite of "doing mode." Instead of trying to fix or change difficult emotions, activating being mode means simply accepting them and allowing them to be.

Do you ever try to "fix" or "solve" certain emotions? If so, how?

How does activating "doing mode" in this way work out for you?

How does constantly focusing on the gap between where you are and where you want to be make you feel?

What does it feel like to simply be, without needing to fix or solve anything?

How does your world change when you observe rather than interpret?

What helps you shift from doing to being mode?

Think of difficult emotions as the weather. You can't stop, fix, or deny rain. It just is.

Turn Off Autopilot

While doing some things on autopilot is convenient, such as brushing your teeth, living with autopilot constantly activated can make you feel separated from life, as if you're looking at things through frosted glass. This tracker will help you to feel more present and engaged.

Day	How did you turn off autopilot?	How did it affect your mood?

How to turn off autopilot:

- Ask yourself, "Where is my mind right now? Is that where I want it?"
- Alter your daily routine.
- Try something totally new.
- Schedule tech blackout times.
- Tune into an autopilot act, such as making a mug of tea. Notice everything.

How did it affect your body?	What did you notice or think?

Your Acting-Up Tracker

Each day for two weeks, note down whether you noticed and changed any anxious behavior (or didn't) and how that made you feel. You can add emotions and colors to the key below.

Day	Did you change your behavior?	How did you feel?
	Y ○ N ○	○ ○ ○ ○ ○ ○ ○ ○ ○
	Y ○ N ○	○ ○ ○ ○ ○ ○ ○ ○ ○
	Y ○ N ○	○ ○ ○ ○ ○ ○ ○ ○ ○
	Y ○ N ○	○ ○ ○ ○ ○ ○ ○ ○ ○
	Y ○ N ○	○ ○ ○ ○ ○ ○ ○ ○ ○
	Y ○ N ○	○ ○ ○ ○ ○ ○ ○ ○ ○
	Y ○ N ○	○ ○ ○ ○ ○ ○ ○ ○ ○

Maybe you were going to respond angrily to an email, but went for a walk until you'd calmed down. Perhaps you switched from doing to being mode and just let your emotions be for a while. Or possibly you went out when your instinct was to cancel—and you had a great time!

Day	Did you change your behavior?	How did you feel?
	Y ◯ N ◯	◯ ◯ ◯ ◯ ◯ ◯ ◯ ◯ ◯
	Y ◯ N ◯	◯ ◯ ◯ ◯ ◯ ◯ ◯ ◯ ◯
	Y ◯ N ◯	◯ ◯ ◯ ◯ ◯ ◯ ◯ ◯ ◯
	Y ◯ N ◯	◯ ◯ ◯ ◯ ◯ ◯ ◯ ◯ ◯
	Y ◯ N ◯	◯ ◯ ◯ ◯ ◯ ◯ ◯ ◯ ◯
	Y ◯ N ◯	◯ ◯ ◯ ◯ ◯ ◯ ◯ ◯ ◯
	Y ◯ N ◯	◯ ◯ ◯ ◯ ◯ ◯ ◯ ◯ ◯

Set a 15-minute timer, remove any distractions, and freely write your thoughts on how anxiety affects your behavior. Can you see recurring patterns? What would you like to change? Does your anxious behavior best represent who you are? Feel free to go off on tangents—and to make mistakes!

Reflect

Which habits of yours make you feel safe but actually hold you back?

How do you feel about your instinctive responses to challenging events—how you instantly want to behave—versus your more considered reactions?

How do self-defeating behaviors make you feel about yourself?

How determined are you to make changes, and what will you put in place to help?

....

....

....

....

....

....

Which character traits currently hidden by unhelpful behaviors are you looking forward to expressing more fully?

....

....

....

....

....

What would your life look like if you could change your anxious behavior?

....

....

....

....

How do you rate your ability to cope with your anxiety now on a scale of 1 to 10?

○ 1 ○ 2 ○ 3 ○ 4 ○ 5 ○ 6 ○ 7 ○ 8 ○ 9 ○ 10

PART FIVE

Own Your Future Calm

Nobody has a working crystal ball. Everyone will make mistakes, and life will inevitably skew off course sometimes. Learning to live with this uncertainty—and accepting that these things will happen—means you can absolutely cope when they do.

Accepting Uncertainty

Do you accept uncertainty as an inevitable part of life, or do you usually do everything in your control to try to eliminate it?

When does uncertainty feel positive to you?

When is a recent time that uncertainty led to something great?

How do you usually try to control situations that are uncertain?

What illusions of control have you outgrown? Do you feel better or worse because of that?

What parts of your personality flourish in uncertain situations?

What long-term goal are you avoiding because you can't predict how it will turn out?

Which best describes how you feel about an uncertain outcome?

Overwhelmed	Worried	Uneasy	Cautiously open	Hopeful	Excited
○	○	○	○	○	○

Which best describes how you act in response?

Freeze or withdraw	Avoid	Wait and watch	Seek info	Make plans	Act fast
○	○	○	○	○	○

In which areas of life are you better or worse at handling uncertainty?

Which of these thoughts best represents how you feel about uncertainty? (You can write your own thoughts into the empty bubble if you like.)

"I hate this. I need closure."

"It's exciting!"

"What will be, will be."

"I can tolerate not knowing if I plan around it."

....

....

....

....

....

....

The Guilt and Shame Spiral

Guilt is the uncomfortable feeling that you've done something wrong or behaved in ways that don't align with your values. Healthy guilt leads to growth and repair. Unhealthy guilt shows up when no change is needed, such as feeling guilty for building personal boundaries.

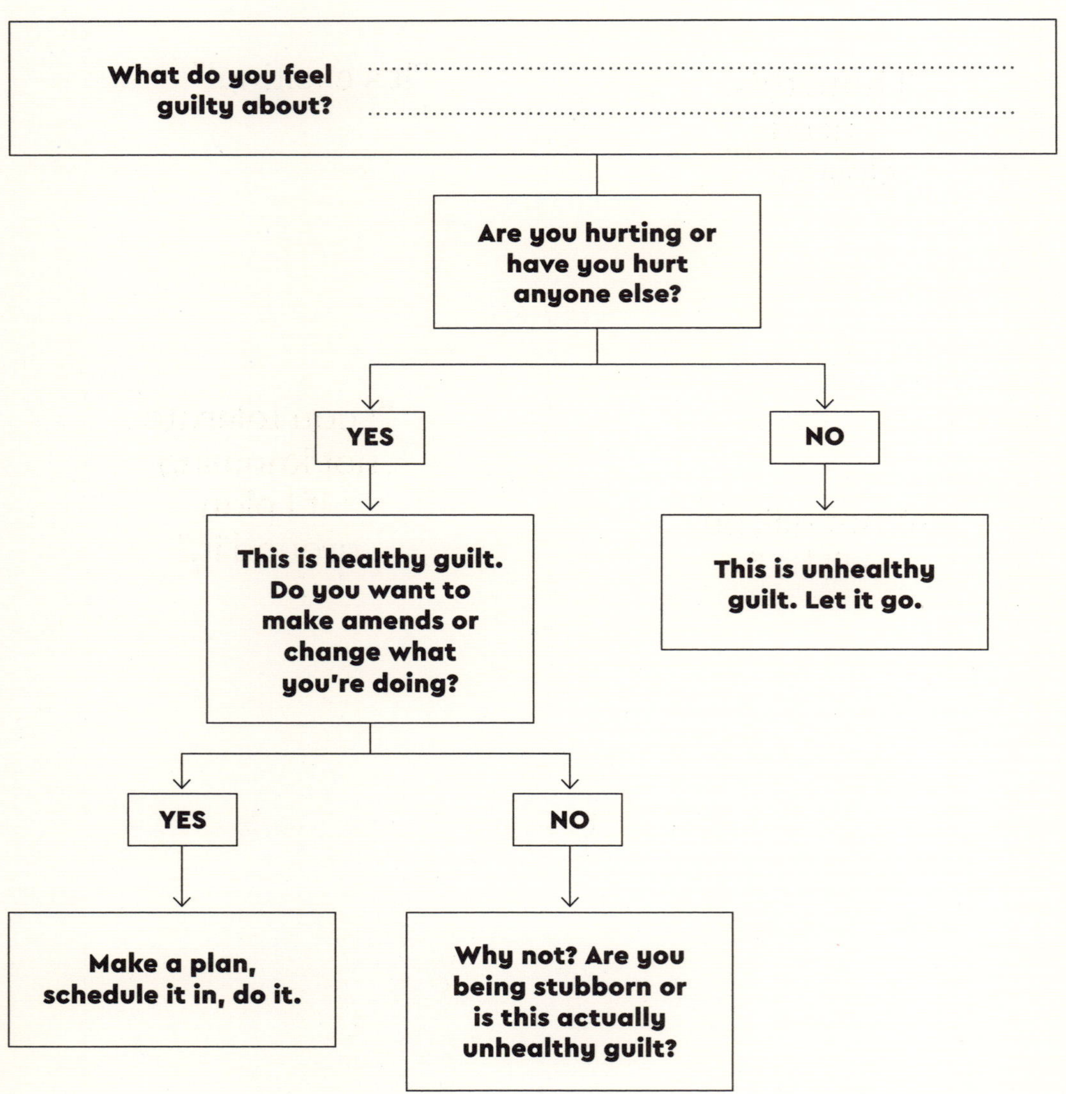

While guilt is about what you did, shame is about who you are. So not, "I did something wrong," but, "I am wrong at my core." Feeling ashamed doesn't mean you've done something shameful! Your inner critic can make you feel ashamed whenever you feel you don't measure up.

When you might feel ashamed:

- When you believe you've failed
- When you receive negative attention, or no attention
- When you act in ways that go against your core values

Why might holding onto shame sometimes feel helpful? For example, when it makes you feel in control.

....

....

....

....

If you turn toward shame rather than running from it, how does it make you feel?

....

....

....

....

Delegation Station

Streamlining your day-to-day will go a long way to easing the anxiety that comes from feeling overwhelmed. Fill in this tracker with your to-do list and work your way through the questions to find tasks that can be delegated or deleted.

What's in your schedule?	How essential is it? (1-10?)	Do it?	Delegate it?	Delete it?

What surprised you from filling out the table?

Are any of these tasks "essential" due to self-imposed "rules" or high personal expectations? ◯ Y ◯ N

Do you assume others will judge you for doing or not doing some of these things? ◯ Y ◯ N

Having a second look now, are there any "do it" things that can be moved into a different column?

Some tasks may take up valuable time, but make you feel good—perhaps calmer or more productive. Fill in this tracker for any that fall into that camp.

Something that takes up time but that you feel is worth it	How it makes you feel emotionally	How it makes you feel physically	What it makes you think	Why it's worth it

And finally, try filling in this last tracker to identify the tasks that have a negative impact. Are these actually essential or can you find a way to delete or delegate?

Something that takes up time and isn't worth it	How it makes you feel emotionally	How it makes you feel physically	What it makes you think	Why it's not worth it

Self-care means taking the time to get to know yourself better.

Self-Care Aware

What does self-care mean to you?

What categories of self-care do you invest the most time and energy in: physical, emotional, mental, social, or spiritual?

Which categories do you want to invest more time in and why?

When it comes to physical self-care, how do you look after yourself?

How does neglecting this affect you?

How do you look after yourself emotionally and mentally?

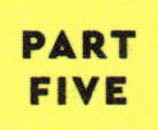

How will you manage any guilty feelings, or reassess any internal rules you have around resting?

What social self-care can you implement? For example, spending more time with loved ones or asking for help when you need it.

What spiritual self-care appeals to you? For example, spending more time in nature.

Your Tough Day Diary

What happened?

....

....

....

....

....

....

How did you feel emotionally at the time?	Note the intensity
....	1 2 3 4 5 6 7 8 9 10
....	1 2 3 4 5 6 7 8 9 10
....	1 2 3 4 5 6 7 8 9 10
....	1 2 3 4 5 6 7 8 9 10

What thoughts were most prominent at the time?

....

....

....

....

....

....

How true were those thoughts?

....

....

....

....

....

How do you feel about it now some time has passed?	Note the intensity
....	1 2 3 4 5 6 7 8 9 10
....	1 2 3 4 5 6 7 8 9 10
....	1 2 3 4 5 6 7 8 9 10
....	1 2 3 4 5 6 7 8 9 10

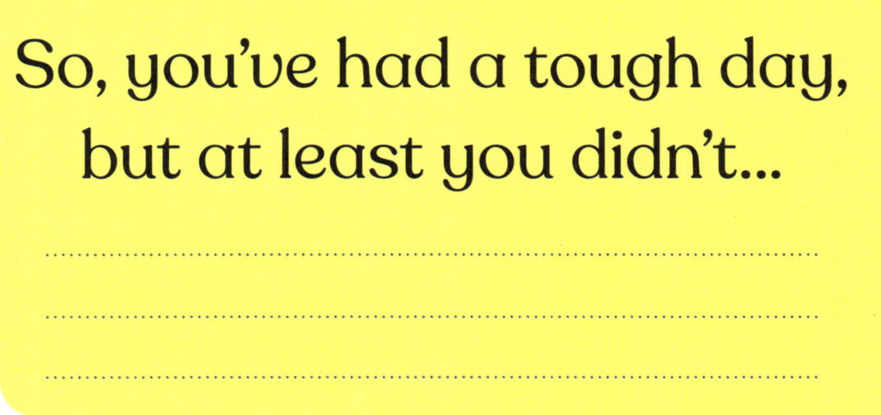

The Clarity Compass

Use this page as your clarity compass when you're spiraling. Work through the questions to travel down the path toward calm, and away from chaos.

When you feel anxious, how else do you often feel?
For example, tired, frustrated, or bored?

....

....

....

....

Who or what can support you?

....

....

....

When and how can you ask for help?

....

....

....

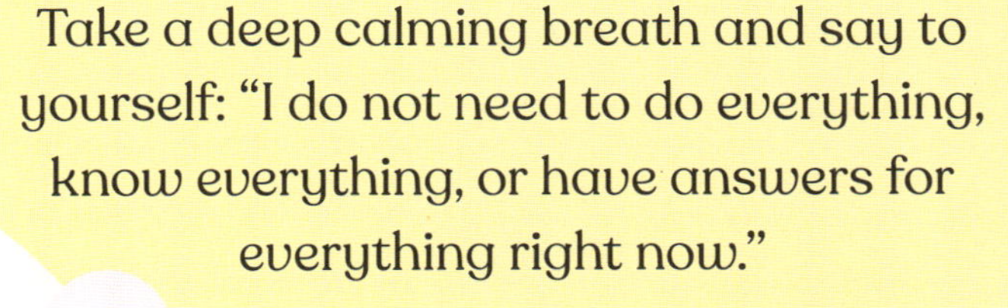

Take a deep calming breath and say to yourself: “I do not need to do everything, know everything, or have answers for everything right now.”

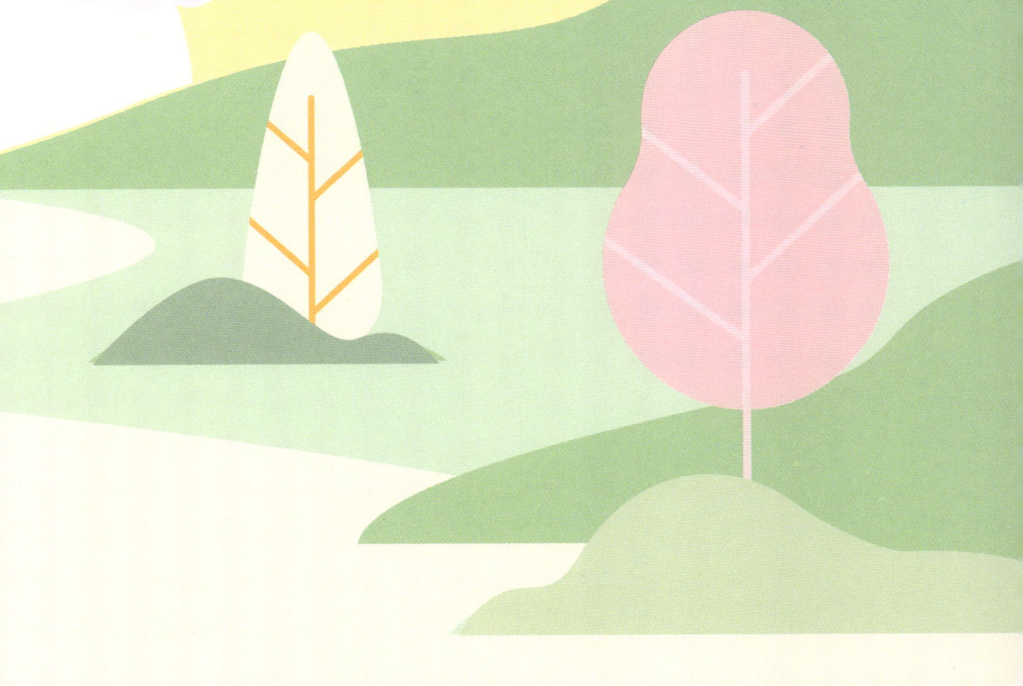

What one small action can you take now to feel calmer?

....

....

....

....

....

....

Positive Speaking

The words you use when you talk to yourself matter. Changing up your vocabulary when it comes to anxiety is a smart way of looking at things differently and challenging negative beliefs.

Instead of "risk" —> Say "opportunity," "chance," "adventure"

Think of a recent time when you called something a risk. How might it have actually been an opportunity?

Instead of "never" and "always" —> Say "sometimes, "often"

What's something you say "always" or "never" happens, but that actually just occurs more or less often than you'd like?

Instead of "should/shouldn't" and "must/mustn't" —>
Say "would/wouldn't," "will/won't," "could/couldn't"

Think of a time when you were hard on yourself. Can you reword the thought using "would" or "will" instead? For example: "I would have liked to handle that differently. I will next time."

....

....

....

....

Instead of "confrontation" and "argument" —>
Say "conversation," "discussion," "exchange"

When did you avoid speaking up because you were afraid of a "confrontation"? Might it have ended up being a "conversation" instead?

....

....

....

Choosing different words may feel like a small thing, but it reflects a big change of mindset—channeling growth and empathy rather than feeling stuck and frustrated.

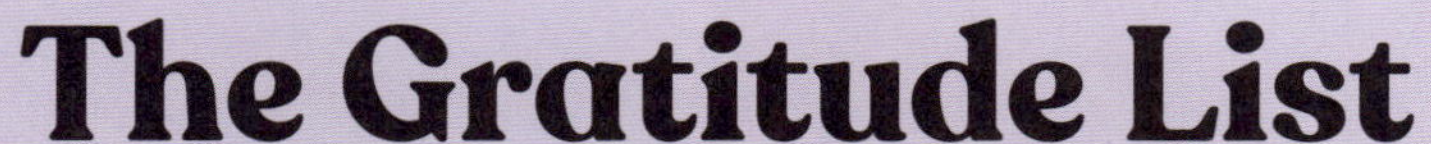

The Gratitude List

Taking stock of what you're thankful for shifts focus from worries onto the good things in life. List some of the things you're grateful for here, big or small. For example, "my friends," "a great book," or "the amazing bakery down the street."

Name one thing that happened today that you're grateful for, big or small.

Who are you particularly thankful for right now, and why?

Name one thing that you achieved or overcame today.

How does thinking about gratitude make you feel emotionally and physically?

Nurture Self-Compassion

Nurturing compassion for yourself is an incredibly important part of learning to own your calm. It means being kind and fair to yourself—and to do that effectively you have to admit that often you're not.

Ask yourself:

1. Would you speak to anyone else the way your inner critic speaks to you?
2. Would you try to motivate someone by chastising them, or by encouraging them in a way that builds trust, confidence, and hope?

Write down something harsh your inner critic said to you recently. Then rewrite it from the perspective of a loving and kind voice.

List parts of your life where your inner critic speaks the loudest. Next to each, write a compassionate message you can remind yourself of next time.

Challenging area	Compassionate response

Self-compassion isn't about letting yourself off the hook. It's about being fair and kind.

Reflect

How has uncertainty in life shaped your personal growth and resilience?

What helps you to feel grounded when you don't know what's going to happen?

How are you going to be kinder and fairer to yourself? Think about self-compassion, self-care, delegating tasks, and more!

When you feel calm slipping away, how are you going to coax it back?

What are some things you can commit to doing for yourself every day?

How do you rate your ability to cope with your anxiety now on a scale of 1 to 10?

○ 1 ○ 2 ○ 3 ○ 4 ○ 5 ○ 6 ○ 7 ○ 8 ○ 9 ○ 10

PART SIX

The Monthly Trackers

Welcome to your twelve monthly mood trackers. At the start of each month, set out your plans, priorities, and hopes for the weeks ahead. As the month unfolds, use the tracker to monitor how you're feeling. Then, at the end of the month, you'll find space to reflect on how things went and why.

HOW DO MOOD TRACKERS WORK?

Getting into a daily tracking habit will help you notice when you feel your best, when you're doing okay, and when anxiety creeps in—as well as how those moods align with the goals you set at the start. It stops anxiety from feeling all-encompassing, providing reassurance that no emotion is permanent and that you do have moments where you feel on top of your game. From there, you can start working out how to do more of the things that make you feel your best.

Let's Get Tracking

What do you hope to learn about yourself from tracking your mood?

How would you describe your relationship with anxiety right now?

What do you both hope and fear might come up as you begin observing patterns?

What would progress look like for you?

What are two or three aims you'd like to carry with you throughout this process?

How can you remind yourself that this is about awareness, not judgment or perfection?

If you miss an entry, don't be hard on yourself—just start again with a fresh mindset.

Mood-Lifting Mantras

I will be patient
with myself.

I will cut myself
some slack.

I will give myself credit
for facing and
overcoming challenges.

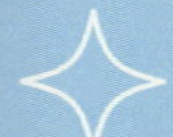

Month One

Fill in this page at the **start** of the month

What is your main focus for this month?

What steps will you put in place to help achieve a sense of calm?

What are you least looking forward to and how can you make it easier?

What are you most looking forward to?

Month One

Fill in this page at the **end** of the month

Note down how you overcame one challenge this month.

Who or what was your biggest support and why?

Which anxiety triggers did you notice most?

When did you feel most calm, strong, and in control?

Monthly Mood Tracker

Fill in the key at the beginning of the month by assigning colors to as many emotions as you like. Then fill in each day with all the key emotions that you felt. Calm can be quiet and so easily drowned out by louder emotions. Try to tune into those softer, more peaceful moments.

○ Calm ○ ○ ○
○ ○ ○ ○
○ ○ ○ ○

1 2 3 4 5 6 7 8 9 10 11 12 13 14 15 16

17 18 19 20 21 22 23 24 25 26 27 28 29 30 31

THOUGHTS AREN'T FACTS

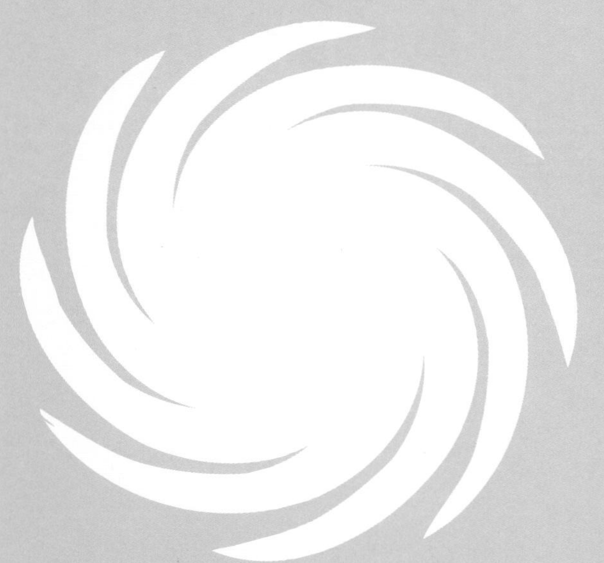

They are just opinions from your biased brain. Accepting that means giving yourself options. Do you want to listen to them? Are they helpful?

Month Two

Fill in this page at the **start** of the month

What calming activities can you make part of your routine this month?

What challenges might you face, and how can you work around them?

What task can you start that you've been putting off or avoiding? Write down the steps you can take to make it seem less daunting.

Month Two

Fill in this page at the **end** of the month

How did any calming activities that you practiced make you feel?

What surprised you about the levels of calm that you noted on the tracker?

Were your avoidance or procrastination tendencies better or worse than last month?

Monthly Mood Tracker

Whenever you feel calm, relaxed, peaceful, or particularly present this month, note down in this tracker what you were doing and who you were with. This can help you see what and who softens anxiety for you.

Day	How I felt	Who I was with	What I was doing	Day	How I felt	Who I was with	What I was doing
1				17			
2				18			
3				19			
4				20			
5				21			
6				22			
7				23			
8				24			
9				25			
10				26			
11				27			
12				28			
13				29			
14				30			
15				31			
16							

"Life is what happens while you are busy making other plans."

– Allen Saunders and John Lennon

Month Three

Fill in this page at the **start** of the month

How will you try to stay present and grounded this month?

How will you rationalize making any mistakes?

What one new thing will you try this month?

Month Three

Fill in this page at the **end** of the month

When, where, and with whom did you feel most calm this month?

What surprised you most after filling in the tracker?

What new thing did you try and how did it go?

Monthly Mood Tracker

Fill in the key at the beginning of the month by assigning colors to as many emotions as you like. Then fill in each day with all the key emotions that you felt. Be mindful that your anxiety may lead you to dismiss "positive" emotions, so, when filling in the tracker, ensure you're giving them equal weight to the tougher ones.

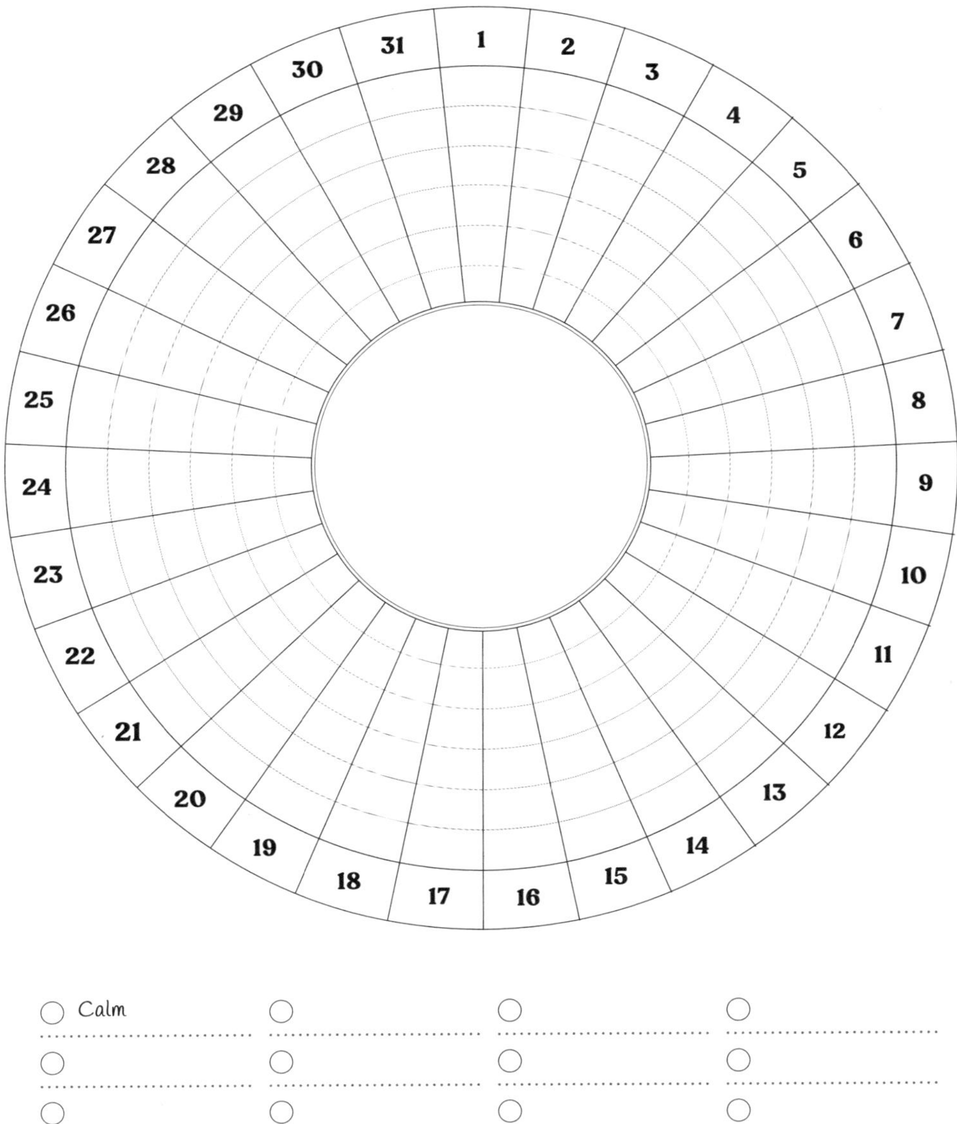

Anxiety is...

An emotion that will pass,
as all emotions do.

A sign your body is trying
to protect you.

A reason to slow down.

A sign you could be stepping
outside your comfort zone
and growing.

Something you can learn
to manage.

A normal part of being human
in an uncertain world.

Month Four

Fill in this page at the **start** of the month

What would make you feel proud this month?

What stressful task can you do, delegate, or delete from your to-do list to make your schedule more calming?

How will you reward yourself for being more self-compassionate this month?

Month Four

Fill in this page at the **end** of the month

Use this space to complete a free-writing exercise reflecting on the past month. Set a timer for 10 minutes and write down everything and anything that comes to mind about how you felt, what went well, what was tough, and how you managed both the highs and lows.

Monthly Mood Tracker

Track three moods and three behaviors throughout the month. Each day, color or check the box if you felt it (mood) or did it (behavior). Choose a range of moods and behaviors—not just the difficult ones. For example, you might track feeling anxious, calm, and confident, as well as behaviors like procrastinating, comparing yourself with others, and practicing self-care.

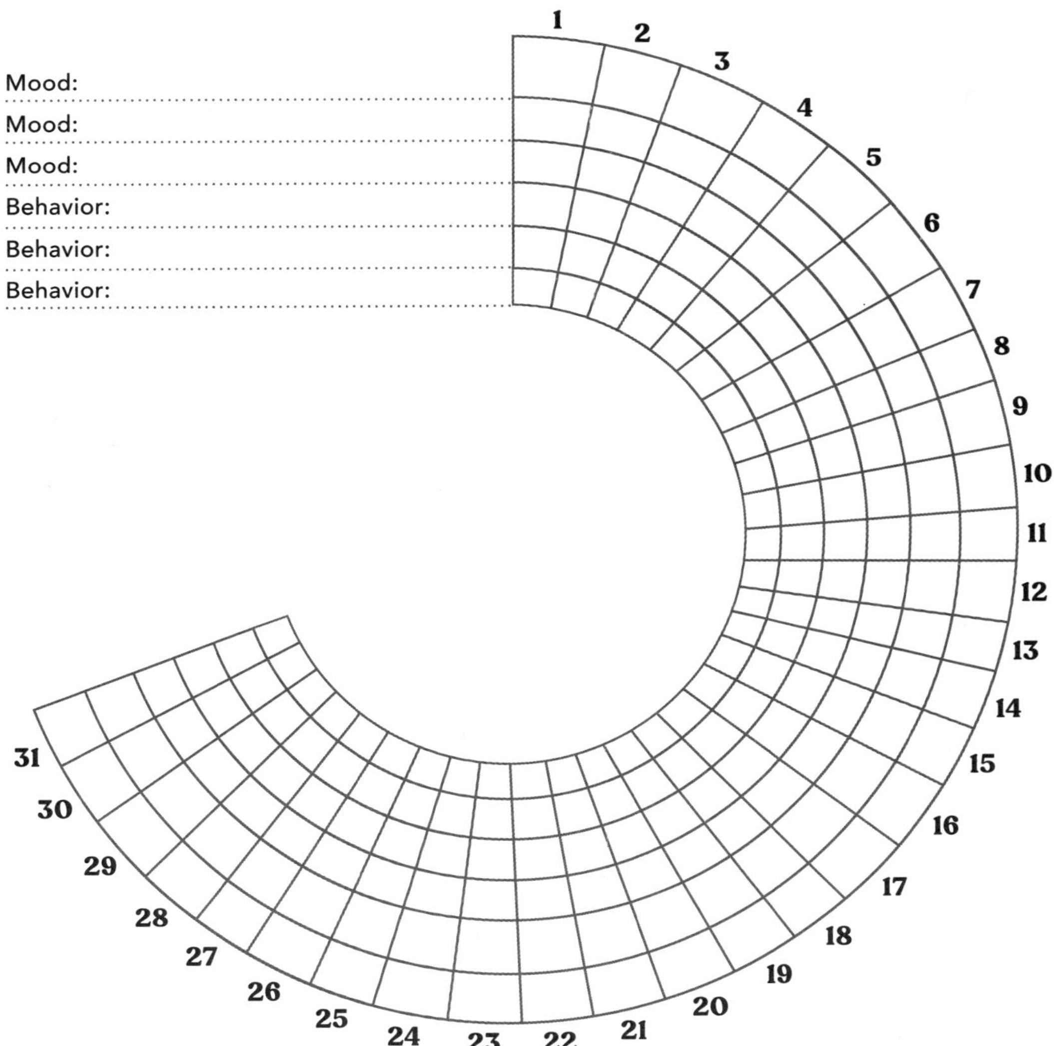

Box Breathing

To begin, sit upright in a chair with your back straight, hands on your knees, and feet firmly planted on the ground. Exhale all of the air from your lungs.

Now, imagine breathing around this box:

1. Inhale slowly through your nose for four seconds, gradually filling your lungs with air.
2. Hold your breath for four seconds.
3. Exhale slowly through your mouth for four seconds.
4. Pause for four seconds.

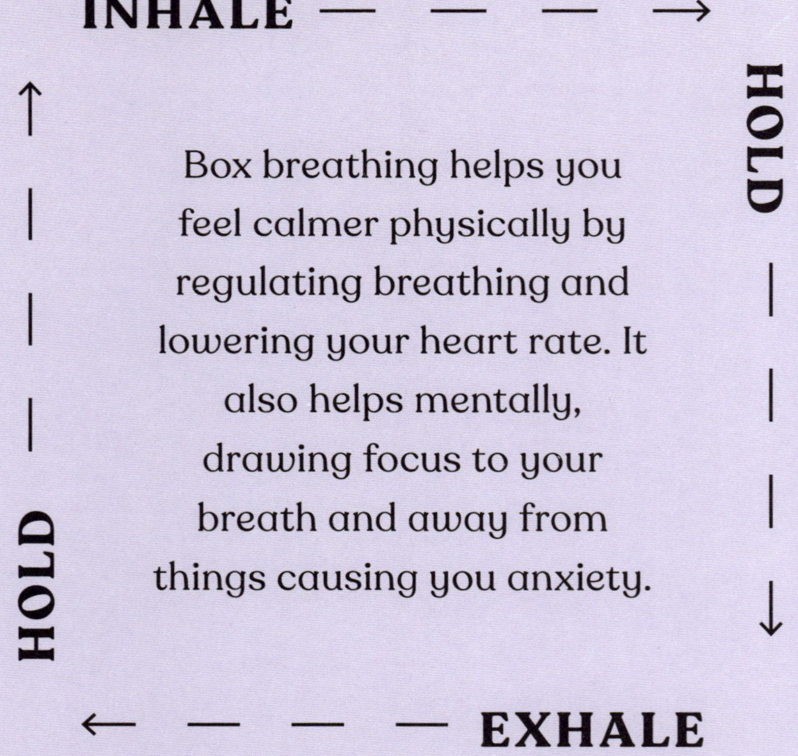

Repeat until you're owning your calm.

Month Five

Fill in this page at the **start** of the month

What lesson (or lessons) did you learn last month that you'd like to carry forward into this one?

What is one goal you'd like to accomplish?

How can you be your own advocate this month?

Month Five

Fill in this page at the **end** of the month

How did you experience anxiety overall this month? Was it less or more than you were expecting, more physical or behavioral, only in certain situations, etc.?

How did you set out to accomplish your goal, and how did it go?

What was surprising or interesting about how you were or weren't your own advocate?

Monthly Mood Tracker

Record each time you do or don't support yourself this month and how it makes you feel. Try to do things that you know will lift your mood, even if you often avoid them, such as listening to music, exercising, eating well, seeing friends, or taking a break.

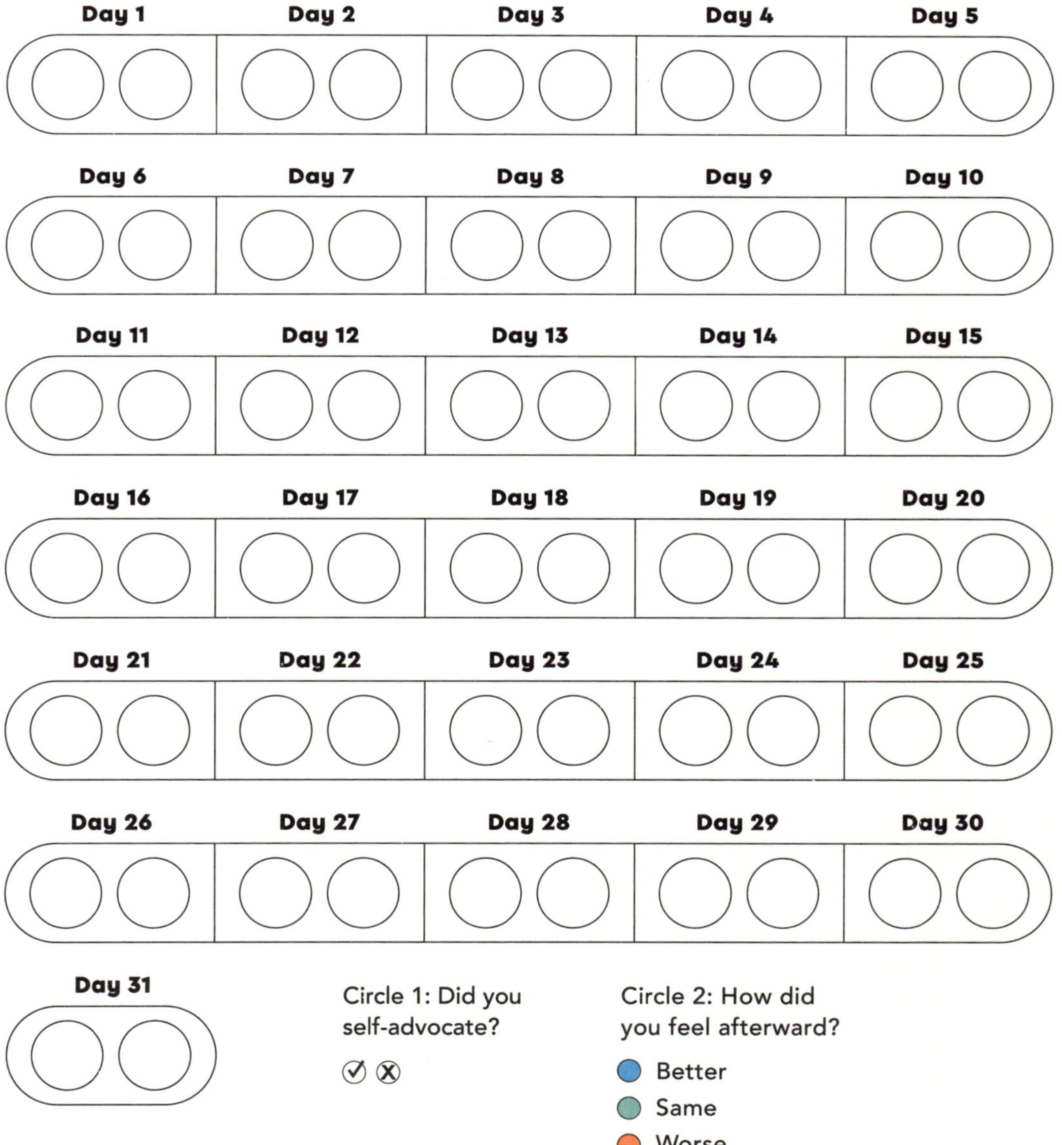

Slow Down the Spiral

Next time you're in an anxiety spiral, ask yourself:

1. "What's the worst that could happen?"

2. "Now, what's the realistic worst that could happen?"

3. "What's most likely to happen?"

4. "What support or tools do I have to help me cope with whatever happens?"

Month Six

Fill in this page at the **start** of the month

Set your intention for this month: What do you want to do and how do you want to feel?

If anxiety wasn't an issue, what is something you would love to try?

Who would you like to spend more time with, or reconnect with, and how can you make that happen?

Month Six

Fill in this page at the **end** of the month

When did you feel your best this month, and why do you think that might be?

What anxious thoughts bothered you the most, and how did you manage them?

Are there any thoughts that you wish you hadn't bothered worrying about because your worst-case scenarios never happened?

Monthly Mood Tracker

At the beginning of the month, fill in the key by assigning colors to the emotions. Then shade each slice of this pie chart with your overarching mood for the day, using gradients or crosshatching to represent how strongly you felt it.

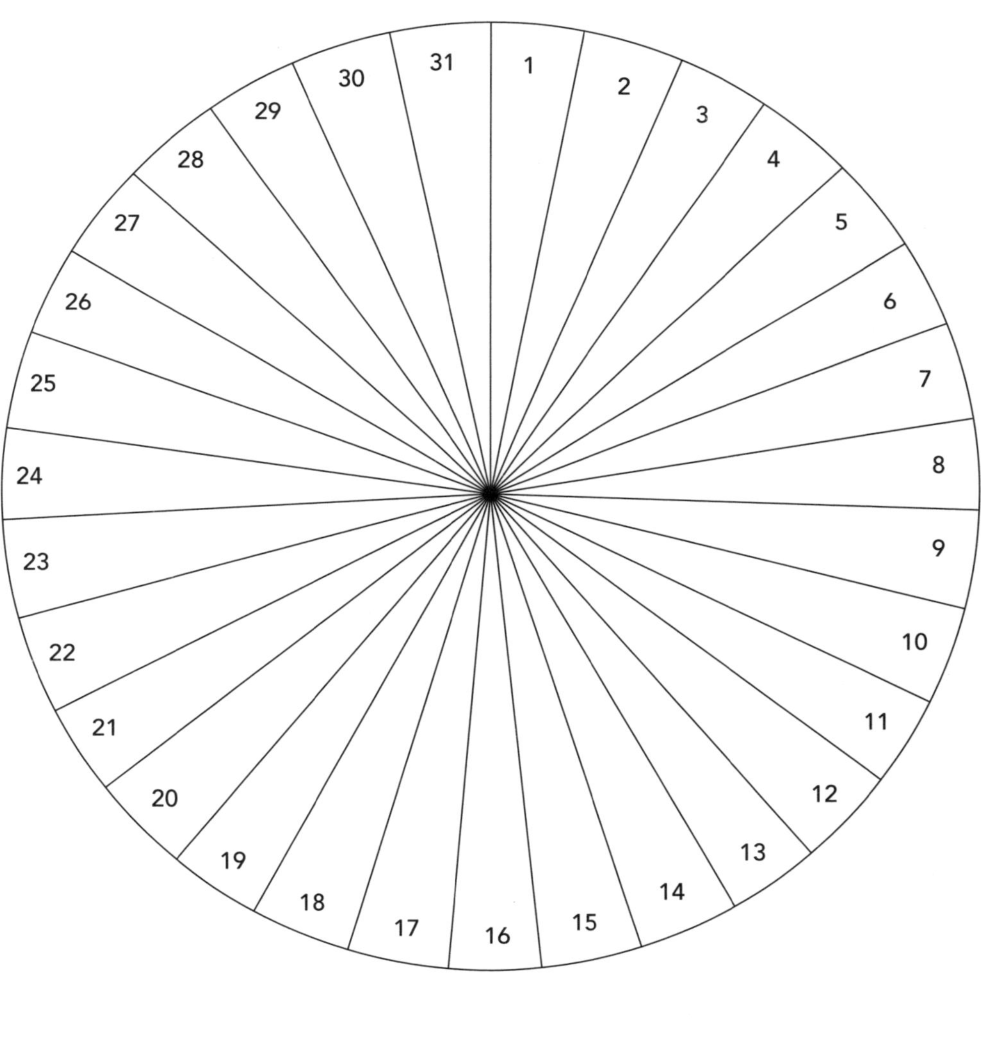

○ Happy ○ Sad ○ Energized ○ ....

○ Calm ○ Angry ○ Neutral ○ ....

Anxiety is not...

A character flaw or measure of your worth.

A prediction of the future.

Always a reflection of truth or reality.

A reason to feel ashamed.

Proof you're unable to cope.

A label or something that defines you. (It's an emotion, not your identity.)

Your fault.

Month Seven

Fill in this page at the **start** of the month

What would feeling emotionally balanced look and feel like for you this month?

Name one overarching intention you want to carry with you this month. For example, "I will treat myself with patience."

What upcoming situations might cause you anxiety this month? How can you prepare for them?

Month Seven

Fill in this page at the **end** of the month

How emotionally balanced did you feel this month?

Did you meet the intention you set at the start of the month?

How did you manage any anxious situations?

Monthly Mood Tracker

This month, track your emotional balance: how calm, collected, and in control you felt each day. You can use either numbers or colors.

Day	Rating (color or number)	Notes	Day	Rating (color or number)	Notes
1			17		
2			18		
3			19		
4			20		
5			21		
6			22		
7			23		
8			24		
9			25		
10			26		
11			27		
12			28		
13			29		
14			30		
15			31		
16					

1 - 2 Very unbalanced (anxious and worried)
3 - 4 Somewhat unbalanced (quite low all-round)
5 - 6 Moderately balanced (some highs and lows)
7 - 8 Mostly balanced (fairly calm and grounded)
9 - 10 Balanced (feeling in control)

“Serenity is not freedom from the storm, but peace amid the storm.”

– S A Jefferson-Wright

Month Eight

Fill in this page at the **start** of the month

What would you like more of in your daily life this month and how will you try to get it? For example, joy, creativity, connection, rest, laughter, and peace.

How can you create a sense of emotional safety for yourself?

How can you soothe yourself when needed?

Month Eight

Fill in this page at the **end** of the month

What moments brought you unexpected calm or joy this month?

What progress did you make, even if it was small or invisible to others?

How will you celebrate this month's wins?

Monthly Mood Tracker

Each day, make a tally mark whenever you experience one of the moments listed. You can mark more than one box per day. At the end of the month, tally up how many times you felt each way. This can help you to be more aware of the moments when you feel peaceful and connected.

Moments of peace, connection, and joy	Did I feel this today? (Use a tally system, so /// = three days)
A proper belly laugh	
A moment of peace and calm	
Feeling connected with myself	
Feeling connected with others	
Creating something freely	
Savoring a simple pleasure	
Breathing deeply and consciously	
I experienced no moments of peace, connection, or joy today	

A Fable

Grandfather:

"Inside me, there are two wolves fighting. One is angry, fearful, anxious, jealous, and full of hate. The other is calm, loving, hopeful, and peaceful."

Grandchild:

"Which wolf wins?"

Grandfather:

"The one you feed."

Month Nine

Fill in this page at the **start** of the month

How can you make time for rest without feeling guilty this month?

What can you forgive yourself for, right now, so you don't carry it into this month?

What's a "win" to aim for that doesn't involve productivity or perfection?

Month Nine

Fill in this page at the **end** of the month

How did you manage any guilt or perfectionism you encountered this month?

What did you tell yourself when you felt bad for taking time out?

How did forgiving yourself for something at the start of the month work out?

Monthly Mood Tracker

Use this wheel to notice moments when you choose self-compassion over self-chastisement. Recognize how positive it is to make mistakes, ease up on self-criticism, and ignore unhealthy guilt. You can add more than one color for each day.

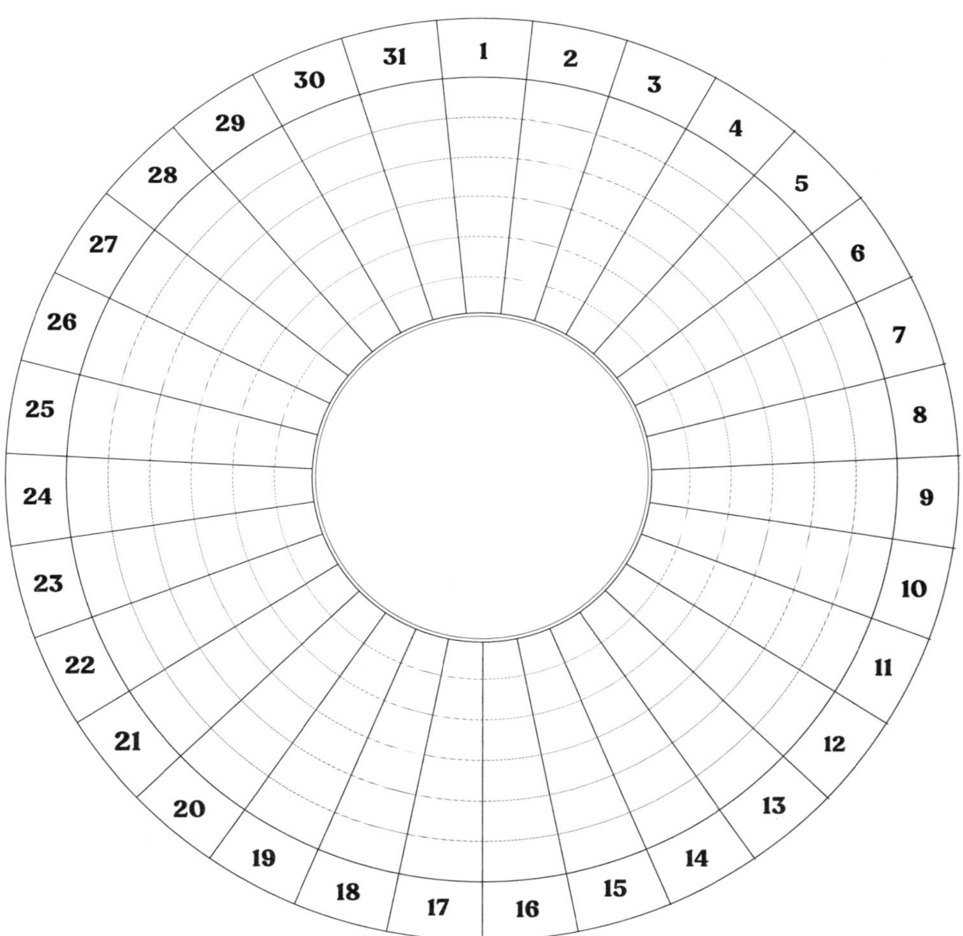

- ○ I was kind to myself
- ○ I forgave myself for something
- ○ I softened self-criticism
- ○ I felt peaceful with imperfection
- ○ I talked myself around from unhealthy guilt
- ○ I didn't get there today, but that's okay

Calm is the emotional equivalent of butter on warm toast: not dramatic or showy, but just as it should be.

Month Ten

Fill in this page at the **start** of the month

What energy or mindset do you want to bring into this month?

What expectations need adjusting to support, not sabotage, your well-being?

What would help you to feel more emotionally steady?

Month Ten

Fill in this page at the **end** of the month

When you felt most anxious, how did you respond?

If you were to speak kindly to yourself about how you handled this month, what would you say?

What habits or anti-anxiety wins do you want to take forward into next month?

Monthly Mood Tracker

Is your glass half empty or half full? This month, bring the classic idiom to life. Each day, mark a line on your glass to show how you felt: the higher the liquid level, the more positive your mood. You can assign colors to specific moods and shade in the liquid too.

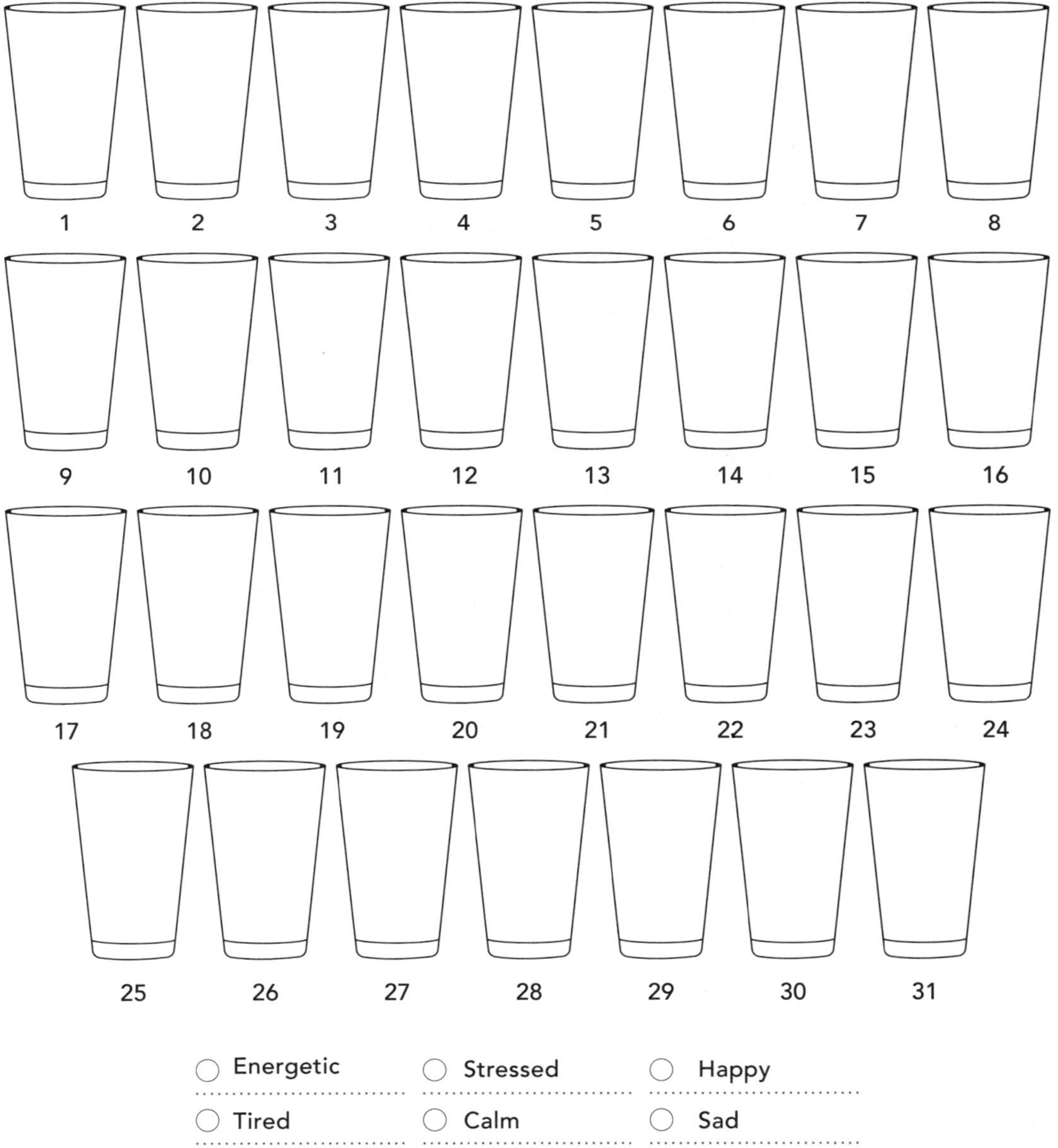

Calm is when neither your mind nor your body is bracing for something.

Month Eleven

Fill in this page at the **start** of the month

How do you want to feel by the end of the month, and how will you try to get there?

How can you prioritize the people or things that make you feel grounded?

What mantra, phrase, or affirmation will you use to guide you this month?

Month Eleven

Fill in this page at the **end** of the month

How did you listen to your energy levels this month?

What truth about yourself do you want to carry into next month?

How did you manage anxiety when it reared its head?

Monthly Mood Tracker

Feeling calm isn't about putting a positive spin on things, but accepting them for what they are. Each day, mark how steady, grounded, and able to cope you felt along the scale. You can make more than one mark if this feeling changed throughout the day.

	Wonky/ Ungrounded	Steady/ Grounded
01		
02		
03		
04		
05		
06		
07		
08		
09		
10		
11		
12		
13		
14		
15		
16		
17		
18		
19		
20		
21		
22		
23		
24		
25		
26		
27		
28		
29		
30		
31		

You deserve
to be here.

Month Twelve

Fill in this page at the **start** of the month

What is one thing that you will do just for yourself this month?

If you treated yourself like someone you cared for deeply, how would that affect what you do?

What are you still holding onto that you don't need to carry into this month?

Month Twelve

Fill in this page at the **end** of the month

What or who brought you comfort this month?

When did you surprise yourself (in a positive way)?

How did you speak to yourself this month? Does that need to change or shift next month?

Monthly Mood Tracker

Each day this month, shade in a puzzle piece with a color to represent the statement that rings most true. (You can use multiple colors for a single piece if more than one happens.)

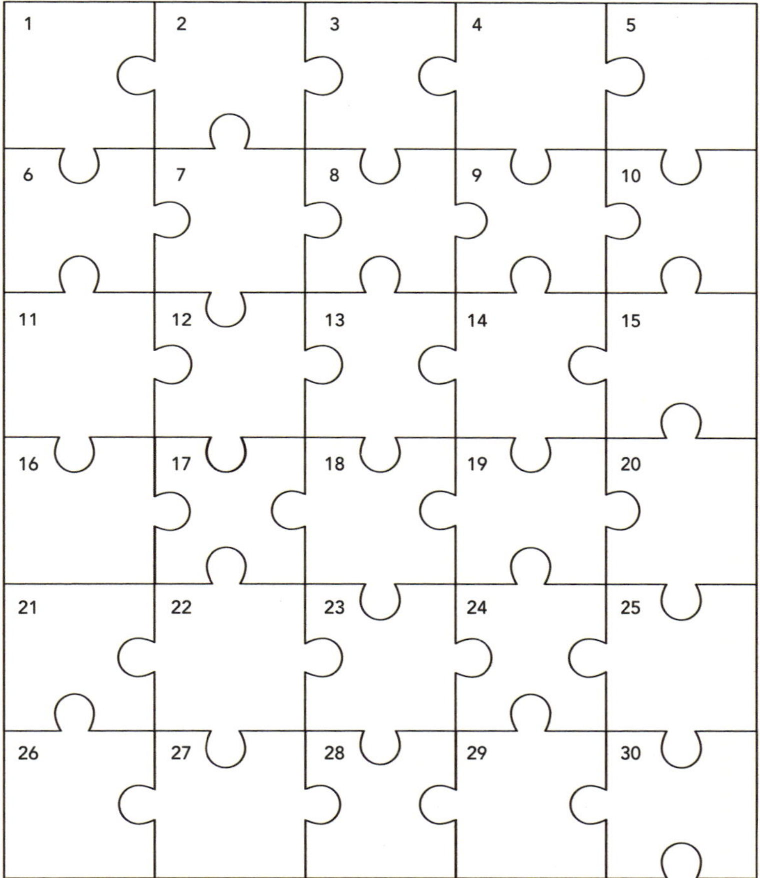

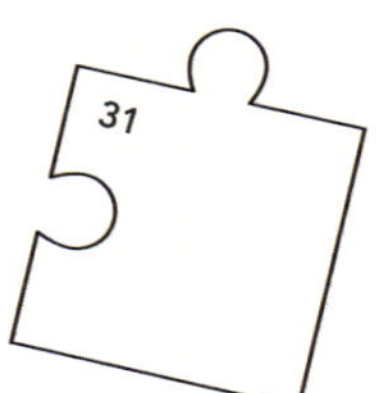

- ◯ I forgave myself for something small
- ◯ I successfully got out of a worry spiral
- ◯ I stopped comparing myself to others or did so fairly
- ◯ I forgave myself for something big
- ◯ I stopped doing something that made me anxious
- ◯ I didn't manage to let anything go today, but can try again tomorrow

Reflect

What patterns or trends did you notice in your mood?

Were there any months or seasons that stood out as easier or harder, and why do you think that might be?

What calming tools or strategies worked best for you? Will you continue using them?

How has your relationship with anxiety changed since you started tracking?

What is the best thing you've learned about yourself throughout this process?

How are you going to reward yourself for getting this far?

How do you rate your ability to cope with your anxiety now on a scale of 1 to 10?

○ 1 ○ 2 ○ 3 ○ 4 ○ 5 ○ 6 ○ 7 ○ 8 ○ 9 ○ 10

Acknowledgments

Jo Usmar is an author, editor, ghostwriter, and journalist. She lives in Amsterdam with her partner, Koen, and their son, Billy.

I would like to thank my brilliant editor Ellie Stores for being so supportive and enthusiastic throughout the writing of this book, as well as Marcia Pedraza Sierra for her beautiful designs. Big thanks to Quarto and Abrams for their willingness to listen to my maddest ideas. This has been a gorgeous project! And, to Koen and Billy, my ports in any storm. You are my calm and my silliness—thank you.

The Bright Press would like to thank Shutterstock for the use of the images used in this book.

Cover © Sasha Balazh, 14 © Egor Shilov, 14 © Aayam 4D, 14 © Foxy Fox, 26 © Fox Design, 35 © KatoSaori, 42 © Pikovit, 51 © Vellot, 56 © mentalmind, 74 © Hanna Olekseichuk, 80 © SanjuBhandari, 86 © Agor2012, 100 © vellot, 112 © Lubo Ivanko, 113 © Martyshova Maria, 144 © Lee Sheng Han, 166 © MOJX Studio, 178 © briddy, 183 © mentalmind, 186 © Molibdenis-Studio, 190 © Olly Kava, 195 © judyjump, 197 © Image Nest, 198 © Elena Pimukova, 202 © Tanya Shulga, 205 © Ekaterina_Zhurina

Every effort has been made to credit the copyright holders of the images used in this book. We apologize for any unintentional omissions or errors and will insert the appropriate acknowledgments to any companies or individuals in subsequent editions of the work.